Coming Into Mind

Contemporary neuroscience has a valuable contribution to make to understanding the mind-brain. *Coming Into Mind* aims to bridge the gap between theory and clinical practice, demonstrating how awareness of the insights gained from neuroscience is essential if the psychological therapies are to maintain scientific integrity in the twenty-first century.

Margaret Wilkinson introduces the clinician to those aspects of neuroscience which are most relevant to their practice, guiding the reader through topics such as memory, brain plasticity, neural connection and the emotional brain. Detailed clinical case studies are included throughout to demonstrate the value of employing the insights of neuroscience. The book focuses on the affect-regulating, relational aspects of therapy that forge new neural pathways through emotional connection, forming the emotional scaffolding that permits the development of mind. Subjects covered include:

- Why neuroscience?
- The early development of the mind-brain
- Un-doing dissociation
- The dreaming mind-brain
- The emergent self

This book succeeds in making cutting-edge research accessible, helping mental health professionals grasp the direct relevance of neuroscience to their practice. It will be of great interest to Jungian analysts, psychoanalysts, psychodynamic psychotherapists and counsellors.

Margaret Wilkinson is an analyst in private practice and an assistant editor of the *Journal of Analytical Psychology*.

Coming Into Mind

The mind-brain relationship: a Jungian clinical perspective

Margaret Wilkinson

To. The Willows Counselling
Service
With best wishes,
Margaret Wilk—
2011

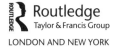 Routledge
Taylor & Francis Group

LONDON AND NEW YORK

First published 2006 by Routledge
27 Church Road, Hove, East Sussex BN3 2FA

Simultaneously published in the USA and Canada
by Routledge
270 Madison Avenue, New York NY 10016

Reprinted 2006, 2007 and 2009

Routledge is an imprint of the Taylor & Francis Group, an Informa business

Typeset in Sabon by RefineCatch Ltd., Bungay, Suffolk
Printed and bound in Great Britain by
TJ International Ltd, Padstow, Cornwall
Paperback cover design by Lisa Dynan

This publication has been produced with paper manufactured
to strict environmental standards and with pulp derived from
sustainable forests.

British Library Cataloguing in Publication Data
A catalogue record for this book is available from the British Library

Library of Congress Cataloging in Publication Data
Wilkinson, Margaret.
    Coming into mind : the mind-brain relationship : A Jungian clinical
perspective / Margaret Wilkinson.
        p. cm.
    Includes bibliographical references and index.
    ISBN 1-58391-708-X (hbk : alk. paper)
    ISBN 1-58391-709-8 (pbk : alk. paper)
    1. Cognitive neuroscience. 2. Cognitive psychology.
    3. Neuropsychology.   I. Title.
    QP360.W53 2006
    612.8'2—dc22   2005023324

ISBN13: 978-1-58391-708-4 (hbk)
ISBN13: 978-1-58391-709-1 (pbk)

Contents

List of figures and plates

Foreword

Psychoanalysis and psychotherapy are now in a dynamic period of growth and change. This acceleration of development in the field of mental health is in large part due to the incorporation of very recent advances in the sciences that border psychoanalysis, clinical psychology, and psychiatry. In particular, a convergence of findings in developmental and affective neuroscience is now enriching and reorganizing fundamental models of early human emotional and social development. The mutually enriching cross-fertilization of knowledge across both the basic and applied sciences has allowed for the creation of more complex psychoneurobiological models of the initial stages of the development of the mind, especially the unconscious mind. These updated developmental advances have in turn generated a deeper understanding of change processes within the unconscious mind that potentially occur over all later stages of the lifespan, including models of change within the psychotherapeutic context.

In a number of recent contributions I am arguing that the interdisciplinary perspective that emerges from the simultaneous and parallel advances in the biological and psychological sciences is acting as a potent catalytic force for a Kuhnian paradigm shift in a number of applied sciences, including psychoanalysis, the science of unconscious processes (Schore 2005a, in press). This current transformation is objectively expressed in a significant increase of clinically relevant interdisciplinary information available to psychotherapists, and subjectively in the amplified energy level within the field. The current dialogue between neurobiological research on the brain and psychoanalytic studies of the mind is thus allowing for a realization of Freud's prediction of a rapprochement between psychoanalysis and the natural sciences (Schore 1997). It is also leading to renewed creativity in re-viewing classic clinical phenomena in light of this fresh psychoneurobiological perspective.

In this timely cutting-edge book Margaret Wilkinson offers an important voice to this interdisciplinary dialogue, effectively demonstrating that recent advances in the sciences that border psychoanalysis need to be incorporated into day-to-day, indeed moment-to-moment therapeutic work. As an exemplary contribution to neuropsychoanalytic scholarship, the author presents the complexity of current neuroscience and developmental data in a clear and understandable fashion, comprehensible and recognizable to clinicians of all schools. A number of current texts are now attempting to bridge the divide between the biological models of the brain and psychological models of the mind. But what particular aspects of human psychology are most relevant to the therapeutic context? Wilkinson's talent, which draws from her extensive clinical experience, is to specifically focus upon intersubjective affective-cognitive mechanisms that operate at the nonconscious core of the psychoanalytic encounter. She then turns to neuroscience to identify the brain systems that structurally mediate these implicit processes.

Written from the pragmatic viewpoint of a working clinician, the early chapters outline clear expositions of current findings in not only neuroscience, but also in development, affect, memory, trauma, and dissociation, areas now of current intense interest to all schools of psychotherapy. At later points of the book she ventures deeply into a topic hardly touched upon in current neuropsychoanalytic writings – adolescence. And in perhaps the most creative chapter (8), she offers an important contribution to psychoanalytic dream work. Throughout all of these applications of neuropsychoanalysis to clinical psychoanalysis, Wilkinson focuses upon recent studies of the early developing right hemisphere, which at all points of the lifespan is dominant for affect processing, implicit memory, the storage of traumatic experiences, and primitive defenses, such as dissociation.

The reader will be enriched by the considerable amount of recent interdisciplinary information provided in these chapters. However, Wilkinson's major contribution is to translate this data into practical clinical material, familiar to psychotherapists, and then to demonstrate the usefulness of very recent advances in developmental, neuropsychoanalytic, and trauma information to more effective work. Knowledge of recent neuroscience may thus inform clinicians about the underlying psychoneurobiological mechanisms that lie at the core of what has previously been referred to as 'internal psychic structure', and how intersubjective processes within the therapeutic alliance transactions facilitate change in these unconscious structures. She boldly asserts that knowledge of current neuroscience can enable clinicians to 'come to a clearer understanding of why they do what they do, especially in relation to the unconscious, empathic, dynamic aspects of work in the transference and countertransference'.

Wilkinson's psychoanalytic perspective of the clinical encounter is significantly influenced by her deep understanding of Carl Jung's analytical psychology. Continuing her earlier seminal publications on the numerous contact points of Jung's writings and the data of contemporary science, this book represents the first detailed exposition of how many of Jung's original psychoanalytic hypotheses, created within the framework of the early twentieth-century science of the unconscious mind, are now validated by neuroscientific findings of twenty-first century neuropsychoanalysis. On that matter, I offer the following thoughts.

In the final chapter of my first book (Schore 1994) I suggested that Jung (1943) described the 'collective unconscious' as an 'image of the world' that is the source of self-sufficiency, as it contains 'all those elements that are necessary for the self-regulation of the psyche as a whole.' The concept of both the self and regulation are, of course, central to Jung's contributions to psychoanalysis. At every stage of the development of his theories Jung returned to the centrality of the concept of the self. This 'innermost nucleus of the psyche' is fundamentally composed of affect experiences, and it acts as a regulating centre that brings about the maturing of the personality. Although he never offered a formal developmental theory of the origin of the self, he was convinced that 'The symbols of the self arise in the depths of the body' (1940). And again, in *Two Essays on Analytical Psychology* (1943) he proposed: 'The self is a quantity that is supraordinate to the conscious ego. It embraces not only the conscious but also the unconscious psyche, and is therefore, so to speak, a personality which we also are'. Indeed, over the course of his writings Jung attempted to shift the focus of psychoanalysis from the ego to the self.

In my own ongoing studies of the origin, function, dysfunction, and repair of the self (Schore 1994, 2003a, 2003b) I have offered a large body of experimental and clinical studies which demonstrate that the implicit self system, formed in the attachment bond of emotional communication between the infant and mother, is located in the early developing right hemisphere. In a conception that echoes Jung's earlier prescient speculations, I have recently concluded:

> Affective processes appear to lie at the core of the self, and due to the intrinsic psychobiological nature of these bodily-based phenomena recent models of human development, from infancy throughout the lifespan, are moving towards brain-mind-body conceptualizations. These models are redefining the essential characteristics of what makes us uniquely human.
>
> (Schore 2003b: xiv)

A growing body of studies now indicates that the early developing right hemisphere (Chiron et al. 1997) is dominant for the emotional and corporeal self (Schore 1994; Devinsky 2000), intersubjective processes (Decety and Chaminade 2003), processing of 'self-related material' (Keenan et al. 2001), self-regulation (Schore 1994; Sullivan and Gratton 2002), empathy (Schore 1994; Perry et al. 2001), mentalizing (Ohnishi et al. 2004), affective theory of mind (Shamay-Tsoory et al. 2005), and indeed for humanness (Mendez and Lim 2004). Furthermore, there is now agreement that 'In most people, the verbal, conscious and serial information processing takes place in the left hemisphere, while the unconscious, nonverbal and emotional information processing mainly takes place in the right hemisphere' (Larsen et al. 2003:).

In other words, neuroscience now confirms that Jung's self system ('the innermost nucleus of the psyche', the 'regulatory centre') and archetypes are processes that are emergent functions of the early developing right brain. In support of Jung's emphasis on self over ego, at the end of a recent volume I concluded: 'The center of psychic life thus shifts from Freud's ego, which he located in the "speech-area on the left-hand side" and the posterior areas of the verbal left hemisphere, to the highest levels of the nonverbal right hemisphere, the locus of the bodily-based self system and the unconscious mind' (Schore 2003b: 270).

Furthermore, in upcoming chapters Wilkinson cites Jung's proposals about an area of previous controversy in psychoanalysis, the relationship of affective processes to trauma. In 1912 he described how the enduring emotional impact of childhood trauma 'remains hidden all along from the patient, so that not reaching consciousness, the emotion never wears itself out, it is never used up' (para.

222). And in 1934, he asserted: 'As a result of some psychic upheaval whole tracts of our being can plunge back into the unconscious and vanish from the surface for years and decades . . . disturbances caused by affects are known technically as phenomena of dissociation, and are indicative of a psychic split' (para. 286). In recent contributions I have suggested that early relational (attachment) trauma specifically impacts the right hemisphere, causing enduring deficits in affect regulation (Schore, 2002), and that dissociation represents an impairment of the vertical cortical-subcortical circuits of the right brain (Schore 2005b, in press). Current neuropsychoanalytic conceptions of psychic structure that Jung described are thus directly relevant to clinical work with the body, archetypal defenses, and affect regulation in treatment of trauma, especially early relational trauma.

Although Wilkinson focuses on Jung's contributions, this informative and thought-provoking volume will be of great interest to therapists of various persuasions, indeed to anyone who is curious about the meanings of the recent advances in science for clinical practice. Thus, the paradigm shift is impacting not only on psychoanalysis but also psychotherapists of all schools who are intensely interested in the underlying mechanisms of developmental and therapeutic change. Neuroscience and psychobiology now clearly demonstrate that psychotherapy produces changes in not only mind, but also brain and body. In the author's own words, this integration of neuroscientific data and psychodynamic models will lead to a 'resurgence of imaginative, and thoughtful clinical work'. What could be a better outcome of a paradigm shift than that?

References

Chiron, C., Jambaque, I., Nabbout, R., Lounes, R., Syrota, A., and Dulac, O. (1997) 'The right brain hemisphere is dominant in human infants', *Brain*, 120: 1057–65.

Decety, J. and Chaminade, T. (2003) 'When the self represents the other: a new cognitive neuroscience view on psychological identification', *Consciousness and Cognition*, 12: 577–96.

Devinsky, O. (2000) 'Right cerebral hemispheric dominance for a sense of corporeal and emotional self', *Epilepsy & Behavior*, 1: 60–73.

Jung, C.G. (1912) 'The theory of psychoanalysis', *Collected Works 4*, New York: Bollingen Foundation/Princeton University Press.

—— (1934) 'The meaning of psychology for modern man', CW 10.

—— (1940) 'The psychology of the child archetype. CW 9.

—— (1943) 'Two essays on analytical psychology', CW 7.

Keenan, J.P., Nelson, A., O'Connor, M. and Pascual-Leone, A. (2001) 'Self-recognition and the right hemisphere', *Nature*, 409: 305.

Larsen, J.K., Brand, N., Bermond, B. and Hijman, R. (2003) 'Cognitive and emotional characteristics of alexithymia: a review of neurobiological studies', *Journal of Psychosomatic Research*, 54: 533–41.

Mendez, M.F. and Lim, G.T.H. (2004) 'Alterations of the sense of "humanness" in right hemisphere predominant frontotemporal dementia patients', *Cognitive and Behavioral Neurology*, 17: 133–8.

Ohnishi, T., et al. (2004) 'The neural network for the mirror system and mentalizing in normally developed children: an fMRI study', *Neuro-Report*, 15: 1483–7.

Perry, R.J., Rosen, H.R., Kramer, J.H., Beer, J.S., Levenson, R.L. and Miller, B.L. (2001) 'Hemispheric dominance for emotions, empathy, and social behavior: evidence from right and left handers with fronto-temporal dementia', *Neurocase*, 7: 145–60.

Schore, A.N. (1994) *Affect Regulation and the Origin of the Self*, Mahweh, NJ: Erlbaum.

—— (1997) 'A century after Freud's Project: is a rapprochement between psychoanalysis and neurobiology at hand?', *Journal of the American Psychoanalytic Association*, 45: 841–67.

—— (2003a) *Affect Dysregulation and Disorders of the Self*, New York: W.W. Norton.

—— (2003b) *Affect Regulation and the Repair of the Self*, New York: W.W. Norton.

—— (2005) 'Attachment, affect regulation, and the developing right brain: linking developmental neuroscience to pediatrics', *Pediatrics In Review*, 26: 204–11.

—— (2005a, in press) 'A neuropsychoanalytic viewpoint: commentary on paper by Steven H. Knoblauch'. *Psychoanalytic Dialogues*.

—— (2005b, in press) 'Attachment trauma and the developing right brain: origins of pathological dissociation', to be published as a chapter in *Dissociation and Dissociative Disorders: DSM-V and beyond*.

Shamay-Tsoory, S.G., Tomer, R., Berger, B.D., Goldsher, D. and Aharon-Peretz, J. (2005) 'Impaired "affective theory of mind" is associated with right ventromedial prefrontal damage', *Cognitive and Behavioral Neurology*, 18: 55–67.

Sullivan, R.M. and Gratton, A. (2002) 'Prefrontal cortical regulation of hypothalamic-pituitary-adrenal function in the rat and implications for psychopathology: side matters', *Psychoneuroendocrinology*, 27: 99–114.

Allan N. Schore
Department of Psychiatry and Biobehavioral Sciences
David Geffen School of Medicine
University of California At Los Angeles

Acknowledgements

Some sections of this book are based loosely on four of my papers published in the *Journal of Analytical Psychology* between 2001 and 2005 (2001 'His mother tongue: from stuttering to separation, a case history', 46 (2) (Chapters 3 and 9); 2003 'Undoing trauma: contemporary neuroscience – a clinical perspective', 48 (2) (Chapters 3, 5 and 6); 2004 'The mind-brain relationship: the emergent self', 49 (1) (Chapters 2, 3 and 9); 2005 'Undoing dissociation: affective neuroscience – a contemporary Jungian clinical perspective', 50 (4) (Chapters 6 and 9). I am especially grateful to the *Journal of Analytical Psychology* and to Blackwell Press for permission to use my articles listed here.

Some chapters also draw on papers that I presented at the International Association Analytical Psychology Barcelona Congress in 2004 and its Proceedings (Chapter 6), the British Association of Counsellors and Psychotherapists' Conference 2004 (Chapter 1), the Hilda Kirsch Children's Clinic Los Angeles Twenty-fifth Anniversary Lectures 2004 (Chapter 3) and the *Journal of Analytical Psychology* Fiftieth Anniversary Conference in 2005 and its Proceedings (Chapter 8).

All of biographical case material presented is in what Gabbard (2000: 1073) has termed 'thick disguise' in order to preserve confidentiality; some case histories may be composites, containing material drawn from several patients.

This book would never have been written without the editorial advice that Barbara Wharton, then co-editor of the *Journal of Analytical Psychology*, gave me when I first submitted an article for publication. I am deeply indebted to Allan Schore for the advice and suggestions he has given to me. I have also benefited from generous advice and encouragement from JoAnn Culbert-Koehn, Chris Driver, Tim and Katie Kendall, Jean Knox, Joy Schaverien, Lenore

Terr, Sandy Walline and Judith Woodhead. I am grateful to Miranda Davies for her thoughtful comments and her permission to include our discussion of material concerning 'Jay' that she presented at the *Journal of Analytical Psychology* Prague Conference in 2001, which was published in the *Journal of Analytical Psychology* in 2002. I am especially grateful to Wendy Hindle and Pramila Bennet for their willingness to help with the preparation and checking of the text before submission for publication. I have also valued the encouragement and advice generously given by Kate Hawes and Claire Lipscomb of Routledge. I would like to thank those people whose case material and art work are included in this book with their permission. These are acknowledgements which are both personal and professional.

I write as a clinician rather than a scientist. My interest is in the history of ideas; the application of these particular ideas to our work in the consulting-room I find ever more powerful. I wish to acknowledge the huge debt that the analytic world owes to the work of Allan Schore, who has brought the attention of many of us to the value of contemporary neuroscience for a better understanding of our analytic practice.

Permissions acknowledgements for figures and plates

Figures

Figure 2.1 from Carter, R. (2000) *Mapping the Mind*, London: Weidenfeld and Nicolson, a division of The Orion Publishing Group.

Figure 2.2 from Gerhardt, S. (2004) *Why Love Matters*, London: Brunner-Routledge.

Figure 2.3 from Edelman, G.M. and Tononi, G. (2000) *Consciousness: How matter becomes imagination*, London: Penguin.

Figure 3.1 from Carter, R. (2000) *Mapping the Mind*, London: Phoenix, Weidenfeld and Nicolson, a division of The Orion Publishing Group.

Figure 5.1 from Gerhardt, S. (2004) *Why Love Matters*, London: Brunner-Routledge.

Plates

Holly's paintings: Plates 1, 2 and 3
Sophie's paintings: Plates 4, 5, 6, 7, 8 and 9

List of abbreviations

ACTH	adrenal corticotrophic hormone
CAT	computerized axial tomogram
CRF	corticotrophin releasing factor
DID	dissociative identity disorder
DSM-IV	*Diagnostic and Statistical Manual of Mental Disorders*, 4th edition
EEG	electro-encephalogram
EMDR	Eye Movement Desensitization and Reprocessing
fMRI	functional magnetic resonance imaging
GABA	gamma-aminobutyric acid
ICD-10	International Classification of Diseases
MDMA	methylenedioxymeth-amphetamine
MPFC	medial prefrontal cortex
MRI	magnetic resonance imaging
NPS	Neutral Personality State
NREM	non-rapid eye movement
PET	positron emission topography
PTSD	post-traumatic stress disorder
REM	rapid eye movement
RIGS	representations of interactions that have been generalized
TMS	transcranial magnetic stimulation
TPS	Traumatic Personality State

Chapter 1

Why neuroscience?

Coming fully into mind is for so many a task still to be accomplished when they come into therapy because early distress or trauma has hindered that process, or difficult relational experience has left it incomplete with developmental milestones not yet successfully negotiated. But what is mind? Is it merely the brain at work? Not so. In the 1990s, 'the decade of the brain', new research tools enabled more detailed knowledge of brain processes. Gone forever are the unquestioning days of the dualism of Descartes, when mind and brain could be understood as two entirely separate entities and scholars of one would not have been expected to be acquainted with the scholarship of those who studied the other. Neuroscientists such as Panksepp have become aware that 'we shall not really understand the brain and the nature of consciousness until we begin to take emotional feelings more seriously, as internally experienced neuro-symbolic SELF-referenced representations' (Panksepp 1998: 339). Edelman and Tononi (2000) pause at the beginning of their discussion of consciousness, how matter becomes imagination, to reflect that

> No matter how accurate the description of physical processes underlying it, it is hard to conceive how the words of subjective experience – the seeing of blue and the feeling of warmth – springs out of mere physical events. And yet in an age in which brain imaging, general anaesthesia, and neurosurgery are becoming commonplace, we are aware that the world of consciousness depends all too closely on the delicate workings of the brain.
>
> (Edelman and Tononi 2000: 2)

As neuroscientists still have to come to terms with the emergence of subjective experience, of consciousness and of mind, so those of us whose engagement is with the mind still need to come to terms with the significance of 'the decade of the brain' for our own thought and work.

While we may acknowledge that radical change has taken place in the study of the mind-brain-body, we might still ask, 'How much do we have to take on board; indeed is it necessary to take any of it on board at all?' From a philosopher's viewpoint Churchland (2002) argues that philosophy cannot afford to ignore neurobiology because at every level, from neurochemicals to cells, and onwards to circuits and systems levels, brain research has produced results bearing on the nature of the mind. There are colleagues who argue that it is not necessary, or that it is too difficult to allow analytic theory and practice to 'come of age', to allow it to move into the twenty-first century so that it may become grounded in the science of our day, some indeed will even argue strongly that it is not desirable. It was not so in the beginning: Freud, Josef Breuer and Jung all studied in Paris with Jean-Martin Charcot, 'the father of neurology'. Freud, the scientist, was at the cutting edge of research in 1896 with his hypothesis that brain cells communicate with one another across spaces that he called 'contact barriers' and Charles Sherrington, a year later, termed 'synapses'. Both Jung and Freud continued to lead thought concerning the conscious and unconscious and concerning the processes of memory, especially those of repression and dissociation. Jung expressed the frustration of this early period of brain research when, in 1935 in his Tavistock Lectures, he commented that the unconscious had to be deduced introspectively and proposed hypothetically. He described consciousness as 'a surface or skin upon a vast unconscious area of unknown extent' and concluded that 'we ought to have a laboratory in which we could establish by objective methods how things really are when in an unconscious condition' (Jung 1935/1976: para. 12, cited in Ekstrom 2004: 661). Jung's dream is now almost within reach with the new technologies that have become available to us. For Jung the unconscious could be divided into two layers, the personal and the collective. Jung's idea of the unconscious also embraced that which had become dissociated, often as a result of early trauma. In building on the work of Pierre Janet and Charcot, he laid the foundations for the links that contemporary Jungians are now able to make into the work of those neuroscientists who concern themselves with trauma theory today and who draw on those very same roots.

Recent developments in the field of neuroscience have achieved what Freud predicted would one day be the case: for the first time science has begun to be able to provide a scientific understanding of why we do what we do in the consulting-room. This in turn is leading to a whole new era of evidence-based research that will become available for us to explore as clinicians. Since the mid-1990s, Schore and Solms have led the analytic world in its thinking about the relation between the two with their separate ground-breaking attempts to explore the Freudian view of the mind in relation to knowledge emerging from the field of neuroscience. Schore, Siegel and Stern have enriched our understanding of the healthy development of the brain and mind in the early years of life.

From the field of infant research and infant observation it has become clear that the unfolding of mind, and the development of self-awareness, is an essentially relational process. These processes are so early and so fundamental to our ways of being that the focus of much psychoanalytic thought has moved from a preoccupation with Freud's ego to thinking that explores the nature of self and self-states. I believe this shift is of fundamental importance for the analytic world and the development of this new thinking is underpinned by the work of neuroscientists such as Damasio, Panksepp and Schore. I find that in many ways much of the new thinking actually revisits much that is explored in Jung's thought about the mind, the human condition, and in particular the self, revealing his thought perhaps to be the most compatible with the insights that are emerging from neuroscience today.

My contention is that in response to the earliest relational experience with the primary care-giver, developing self and mind arises out of the developing brain, these in turn affect the brain's development as new neural connections are made as a result of interactions with significant others throughout life and not least within the consulting-room. The significance for the work of therapy is immediately apparent. Changes will occur in the configurations of both mind and brain in client and in therapist as new neural connections are made as a result of their interactions.

Thus the initial development of mind is relational and associative, the product of inner and outer experience, arising from the earliest experiences of relationship encountered in the experience with the primary care-giver. Panksepp, Schore, Trevarthen and many others emphasize that both development of mind and genetic expression are experience dependent. They stress the relational, intersubjective nature of the development of the individual self. The richness of the insights that have emerged from the work of Winnicott, Bowlby, Ainsworth and the attachment theorists integrate seamlessly with the work of Panksepp and Schore.

Several years ago, and before I began my exploration of neuroscience, a group of trainees just about to qualify asked me if I would come and speak to them about the most important influences on my analytic practice. As I considered the question I was almost surprised to find, after my own analysis, training and patients, how highly I valued the detailed observation of a child from birth to 2 years of age, undertaken in the late 1970s as an optional part of my training. I realized that it was because it had enabled me to appreciate, long before the plethora of reading about attachment and about neurobiological understanding of the early development of the human mind had become available, how the earliest relation first to mother, then to father and meaningful others, is crucial in the development of a sense of self. It had also helped me to understand the way in which mind develops in relation to other minds. So I would like to introduce you briefly to Jacques, who was a large, fair, first-born baby of a professional couple in their thirties. He remained asleep in his pram throughout our first encounter when he was 6 weeks old. At the time I was struck by his capacity to be aware of his mother as special even in sleep. I observed:

His mother leaned forwards towards the pram. Jacques' eyelids fluttered momentarily then he returned to sleep. His mother could not see this from where she was sitting. A little later she leaned forward to look at him. He immediately stirred, lifted his head slightly, and then buried it in the pram mattress. She had not touched him nor made any sound. His father and I looked into the pram several times but he did not stir for us.

Some research has demonstrated that infants show an attraction for face pattern within the first minutes of life and that by around 8 weeks a baby is able to distinguish his mother's face from other faces (Morton and Johnson 1991). Observing Jacques at 2 months I noted:

His eyes followed his mother as she moved about the room. As his mother went out of the door his eyes came to rest on a painted mask-face of a woman that was on the ledge above the door. He looked at it dreamily and rather sadly. His eyes followed his mother again as she returned and crossed the room. She went out again to fetch the water for his bath. He sat quietly tilting his head upwards at the mask-face. He pursed his mouth and seemed to wrinkle his nose, looking at it with distaste but he continued to gaze at it until his mother returned. His hands were held up in front of him. His eyes met his mother's as she came back through the door. He clasped his hands together momentarily. She smiled down at him. He was looking into her eyes, smiling and gurgling to her. He made slow circling movements with his arms.

Further research notes that studies indicate that the right hemisphere is dominant for face recognition throughout life but also that 2-month-old infants looking at their mother's face appear also to recruit what, in the left hemisphere, will later become their language network. The researchers proposed that 'co-activation of the face and the future language network sustains the facilitative efforts of social interactions, such as looking at the mother's face, on language development' (Tzourio-Mazoyer et al. 2002: 460).

From around 1 year old Jacques' father took more active interest in his management and in the observations. Jacques crawled at 10 months old but did not walk until 15 months when night-feeds had stopped. His father seemed to sense that some further degree of separateness from mother was essential if Jacques were to take his first step and he helped both Jacques and his mother through this difficult transition with sensitivity. He slept in the child's room so that he could rock him to sleep if he woke. His desire for his child to become separate and able to deal with the outside world was symbolized in his gift of a large plastic Rolls-Royce car for him to ride on for his son's first birthday. Yet he also got caught up in a sense of loss for he said with sadness: 'It'll never be the same again will it? Not like his first birthday'.

My observations from long ago are now informed by understanding drawn from attachment theory and from the 'powerful methods and new technologies in neuroscience . . . that are yielding previously undreamed of knowledge about the physiological underpinnings of the inner world' (Solms and Turnbull 2002: 5). My contention in this book is that, while readers may not experience a radical change in what they observe and how they work in the consulting-room, as a result of their acquaintance with neuroscience they may come to a clearer understanding of why they do what they do, especially in relation to the unconscious, empathic, dynamic aspects of work in the transference and countertransference.

It has been widely observed that the period of growth and development of psychoanalytic theory has been marred by the tendency of analysts to generalize from the particular, leading to the fragmentation of the profession into different schools, and groups within groups within those schools. Indeed Fonagy has been moved to comment: 'there is some truth in the quip that analytic clinicians understand the word *data* to be the plural of *anecdote*' (Fonagy 2003: 15, italics in original). I might be accused of doing just that if I had hypothesized merely on the basis of what I had observed with Jacques, rather than relating the observed material to the conclusions of recent empirically based research. Fonagy argues that the failure to link theory to practice in a creative way has been caused by the failure of analytic theory as a scientific theory (Fonagy 2003: 29). It seems that if analytical psychology, indeed psychoanalytic psychotherapy in general, is to survive in the modern world, there is every reason to turn back to the basic principle of our founding fathers, that is to understand, in Jung's words, that 'natural science combines two worlds, the physical and the psychic [and that] psychology does this *only in so far as it is psychophysiology*' (Jung 1946: para. 162, italics mine). It is my contention now that there is much that is worth thoughtful consideration emerging from the field of affective neuroscience, that careful study of it may help to ground our theory and practice more adequately, and that such grounding will enable a resurgence of imaginative, and thoughtful clinical work as we integrate these insights with the rich understanding born of a hundred years of careful clinical work that has taken place right across the wide spectrum of the psychological therapies since Freud's initial observations.

The non-biased, non-subjective measures of outcome so urgently needed by the psychotherapy research of the future will become more possible, as through the use of increasingly sophisticated neuro-imaging techniques, we are able to identify the neural correlates of complex subjective states. However, caution must be exercised in the claims made for such techniques. In experimental work difficulties are encountered that arise from the limitations of the very techniques themselves. These techniques are still in their infancy and much research hitherto has been animal research. The time spans of neuro-imaging consist of milliseconds compared to the time spans involved in the psychotherapeutic process. Canli (2004) stresses the need to design studies that 'can capture the complex interactions between genetic and environmental variables [in order to establish] the behavioural and cognitive mechanisms underlying personality' (Canli 2004: 1125). He urges the need for cooperation between all concerned, from the neuroscientists to those concerned with the psychology of personality. Fonagy believes that scanning techniques that make possible the simultaneous imaging of two individuals interacting may make it possible for us to explore relationship quality as this changes as a consequence of psychotherapy (Fonagy 2004). Solms and Turnbull note that the limited number of functional-imaging studies that have been conducted so far indicate that psychotherapy does indeed change the brain, and that these changes affect the prefrontal lobes (Solms and Turnbull 2002: 288).

Genes we now know are not the code of life *per se* but require environmental stimulus to become activated. Nevertheless, we are becoming aware of the greater propensity of some people to be affected by depression and that this propensity is both genetic and identifiable. Caspi and colleagues' research indicates that for those with a genetic propensity to depression, the likelihood of diagnosis of a major depression in the presence of three or more traumatic life experiences, increases from 10 per cent to 28–32 per cent. In those without this inherited disposition the risk of a major depression is 10–16 per cent regardless of challenging life events (Caspi et al. 2003: 386–9). With such knowledge it becomes possible to identify target groups for treatment.

Green argues that

> a biological approach which takes as a given that the brain is a substrate of mind (while not reducing mind to brain) and can demonstrate its mechanisms and workings, offers us another way of thinking about and understanding what is occurring [in the consulting-room].
>
> (Green 2003: 4)

Green (2003) cites Westen and Gabbard's comment that 'to understand the mechanics of the mind does not mean one has to approach the mind like a mechanic' (Westen and Gabbard 2002: 60). I would suggest we can use the insights arrived at through our understanding of neuroscience to assist us with the creative meaning-making process that is at the heart of good therapeutic endeavour.

The plasticity of the brain is a central concept underpinning the understanding of both the development of mind and nature of the therapeutic cure that is argued in this book. There are sensitive windows of time in the development of both the infant and the adolescent. In the infant the optimum development of circuits in the prefrontal cortex, the early development of mind, is dependent on the quality of the earliest care-giving experience, with significant consequences for the emotional growth of the young mind. Because it is such a vital period of development affecting the way the rest of our experience unfolds Sue Gerhardt's (2004) book *Why Love Matters* has become immensely popular just because she explains this in such an imaginative and accessible way.

In the first three years of life and again in adolescence there is a growth spurt in neural connections in the brain followed by a neural pruning based on the 'use it or lose it' principle. The effect of emotional deprivation in the early years was brought to the attention of us all through the plight of the Romanian orphans. Siegel explains: 'It is the human connections which shape the neural connections from which mind emerges' (Siegel 1999: 2). The plasticity that is such a feature of the adolescent brain may in some ways be a mixed blessing for it is the brain's plasticity that permits programming, that enables the social, emotional and intellectual learning and development characteristics of adolescence, but which also permits pernicious forms of programming such as addiction, whether to alcohol, street drugs or cutting. However, I regard as central to our understanding of how change comes about in analytic work the knowledge that, although emotional growth may be stunted as a result of poor early experience, the plasticity of the brain, and in particular the cerebral cortex, permits the possibility of change throughout life, especially in the context of enabling relationships.

The plasticity of the brain is particularly relevant when we consider the effects of trauma and question how much, if at all, adverse early experience may be undone. In recent years huge interest has developed in contemporary neuroscience and attachment theory and their relevance to the un-doing of trauma (Wilkinson 2003). As Jacques demonstrates, from the beginning the development of mind is dependent on experience of relating to others, the initial development of mind arising from intimate interactions with the mother and also the father. Earliest experiences of emotional states arise out of bodily experiences again in relation to the primary care-giver. The mind-brain-body being that came to be Jacques emerged from the experience of the earliest and most fundamental experiences of relating. Both nature and nurture had a part to play in the growth and development of the neuronal connections that went to make up his individual mind.

Early brain development is adversely affected by traumatic experiences in the earliest relationships. Teicher's (2000) research has shown the impaired connections between right and left hemisphere. In particular, the fibre tract known as the corpus callosum that is the major highway between the two hemispheres may be reduced through the effects of trauma in those who have experienced childhood sexual abuse (Teicher 2000). Schore (2005) has brought together evidence from a substantial body of research, including research using electro-encephalogram (EEG), neuro-imaging (fMRI) data and positron emission topography (PET), that demonstrates that unconscious processing of emotion is associated with the right and not left hemisphere and that the right hemisphere is densely interconnected with limbic regions and therefore contains the major circuitry of emotion regulation. In his most recent writings, Schore stresses the importance of the 'hierarchical vertical corticosubcortical functions' of the right brain and argues that dissociation is best understood not in terms of disconnection of left and right brain but in terms of a loss of connectivity within the right hemisphere (Schore in press).

It is plasticity that enables the change and learning that occurs in therapy. Although the amount of development of new neurons in adulthood is still under debate, the development of new neural pathways is known to be commonplace as synapses change every time we record an experience. It is here that the painstaking work of therapist and client becomes relevant. In particular we might note Levin and Modell's work that shows more brain centres light up in response to metaphor than any other form of human communication, thus indicating the formation of new neural pathways arising from and in response to the symbolic (Levin 1997 and

Modell 1997, cited in Pally 2000: 132). New connections are not created as entirely new entities but rather are added to pre-existing connections. Hebb's (1949) notion that cells that fire together wire together is often used to describe this process.

This process of cure is not only the making of unconscious conscious as with interpretation but also the total interactive experience within both members of the analytic dyad. Through experience within the dyad, new entities are added to pre-existing connections in both brain-minds. Past is revisited at the level of the implicit, changing deeply founded ways of being and behaving then linked with present by means of transformative interpretation within the context of actual relational experience, leading to change in the nature of attachment. This mirroring of healthy early relational experience by the analytic dyad enables the process of affect-regulation, first by the analyst and then by the patient. Therapy is for me rather like a double helix where left brain and right brain processes, one predominantly cognition and the other predominantly affect, intertwine. It is a therapy that pays attention to the present moment, to affect, state and process, not just cognition. This way of working is at the heart of the response of the psychodynamic therapies to the insights that are emerging from affective neuroscience. Interpretations without such grounding are merely cognitive, engaging primarily the left hemisphere. However, I must also emphasize that well-timed interpretations that involve putting feelings into words thus encouraging healthy and integrated functioning of both hemispheres of the brain, must remain an intrinsic part of the process of the coming into mind.

Neuroscientists argue that affectively focused treatment alters the frontal lobes of the brain (Schore 2001a: 315) in a way that is detectable by functional imaging studies (Solms and Turnbull 2002: 288). LeDoux speculates that analysis works by strengthening cortical control over the amygdala (LeDoux 1996: 265), and indeed this is an essential aspect of the analytic process. However, the thesis of this book is that, as Jung knew, such development occurs most effectively when unconscious influences unconscious, changing ways of being and behaving stored deep in implicit memory. Only then can very poor early relational experience which occurred before the emergence of mind, or trauma so severe that it could not remain in mind, be brought fully into mind.

Schore points out that the prefrontal limbic cortex retains the plastic capacities of early development throughout the lifespan thus making possible therapeutic change (Schore 2001b: 73). 'It is the nature of the human brain to store experience – all experience – and to generalize from the specific to the general' (Perry 1999: 20–1). Through the transference relationship with the analyst, the patient is able to explore his or her own deeply established patterns of reacting to another, which are speculatively understood as the expression of activity down neural pathways formed by earlier experience. Through the countertransference the analyst is first able to live them with the patient, then through the analytic process to examine the recurring patterns with the patient. Through the analytic process, new entities are added to pre-existing connections, in the transformative way that is the outcome of appropriate and well-timed interpretation. Schore comments that affectively focused treatment can

> literally alter the orbito-frontal system [of the brain and suggests that the] non-verbal transference-countertransference interactions that take place at preconscious-unconscious levels represent right hemisphere to right hemisphere communications of fast-acting, automatic regulated and dysregulated emotional states between patient and therapist.
>
> (Schore 2001a: 315)

Clinical material is at the heart of this book, showing these insights at work in the consulting-room. I seek to demonstrate the value of the affect-regulating, relational aspects of analytic work that forges new neural pathways through emotional connection. Emotional truth underpins the experience of memory and also the dreaming process as they emerge in the consulting-room, and is confirmed by the analyst's experience in the countertransference. The case material seeks to demonstrate how interactive experience within the analytic dyad enables the development of the emotional scaffolding necessary for the emergence of reflective function, for 'coming into mind'.

Perhaps as yet speculative, nevertheless it may be inferred that the therapeutic process and the evolving symbolizations associated with it can develop new neural pathways in the brain, and in particular can develop the fibre tract known as the corpus callosum that is the major highway between the two hemispheres, shown to be reduced through the effects of trauma (Teicher 2000). It is 'the blending of the strengths of the right and left hemisphere [that] allows for the maximum integration of our cognitive and emotional experience with our inner and outer worlds' (Cozolino 2002: 115). Such integration is facilitated as, through the experience of the transference, past is linked with present and emotional experience revisited and reworked. Siegel comments that 'when one achieves neural integration across the hemispheres one achieves coherent narratives' (Siegel 2003: 15). Analytic work that encompasses relational as well as interpretive agents of change can bring about the integration of the activity of the hemispheres of the mind-brain that then permits the self to emerge more fully through the process of individuation.

Chapter 2

Brain basics

> Natural science combines two worlds, the physical and the psychic.
> Psychology does this only in so far as it is psychophysiology.
>
> (Jung 1946: para. 162)

Looking at the brain

Much of the knowledge about brain structure and functioning that comes to us from contemporary neuroscience has become available because of the development of increasingly sophisticated methods of looking at the brain. Imaging techniques have enabled an understanding of brain structure and function and have identified the location and loci of brain activity, affect stimulation and expression within the brain. The EEG has long been used to measure fluctuations in electrical activity in the brain. More recently the CAT (computerized axial tomogram) scan has made possible the production of a series of X-ray images representing 'slices' of the brain. Recorded signals of the brain's selective take-up of radio waves can also be used to produce the detailed brain images known as MRI (magnetic resonance imaging) scans.

Two further types of scan are beginning to enable neuroscientists to look for changes in the brain while it is actually 'at work'. When a particular part of the brain is active, more oxygen is required, and an fMRI (functional magnetic resonance imaging) scan is able to record and translate this increase in oxygen uptake by haemoglobin into computer images thus recording enhanced activity in specific brain areas. This type of scan is able to scan rapidly and offers the finest resolution of all the scans but is very expensive. The PET scan records and translates into computer images the effects of an injection of a radioactive substance that gives off gamma rays: active areas of the brain appear red. The resolution is less defined and they necessitate a radioactive injection, which limits their use.

It is the development of these 'new non-invasive imaging techniques that allow three-dimensional spatial mapping of metabolic activity (which reflects the level of neuronal activity) in real time' (Sherwood 2005), and in particular the use of fMRI and PET scans, that has enabled much of the advance in neuroscience. In the words of Solms and Turnbull, they are 'yielding previously undreamed of knowledge about the physiological underpinnings of the inner world' (Solms and Turnbull 2002: 5). But some caveats are required when assessing the contribution they can make to our knowledge at present. Imaging techniques cannot yet examine the complexity of interaction between brain regions. The time frames under consideration are those of milliseconds rather than the observational time frame of years in traditional analysis. Equipment remains clumsy, expensive and difficult to access. Much of the research data so far has been based on animal studies although human research data is now beginning to be available. Those who seek to map the brain have become increasingly aware of the complexity of that which they seek to map and, because of this, they are also increasingly aware of the danger of false positives in research results. With these words of caution in mind, I suggest we are experiencing the birth of a new and exciting era in our understanding of the brain-mind.

Cells and their connections

Cells and their connections produce the functioning mind that has for so long been the subject of our detailed observation in the consulting-room. The brain consists of a dense network of cells, many are glial cells that hold the brain together, the building bricks of the structure. The other cells, called neurons, are the ones that do the signalling work that is at the heart of brain activity and that maintains the functioning human being. All neurons have a centre that is able to carry an electrical impulse. Each has dendrites, tendrils that receive messages from other neurons, and axons that transmit the messages to neighbouring cells that fire in their turn. Some cells have short axons designed to reach cells nearby, others have long, thin axons, covered in white myelin (a fatty substance), which enables conduction to the furthest parts of the body; brain cells communicate with one another across spaces (see Figure 2.1).

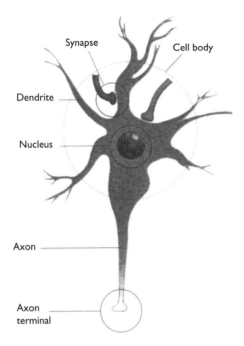

Figure 2.1 A neuron

Source: Carter (2000: 38)

In LeDoux's words, 'Every brain has billions of neurons that together make trillions of synaptic connections among one another' (LeDoux 2002: 49). We are also aware that information transfer within a single neuron is an electrical process, but at synapses the electrical language of the brain is converted into chemical transmitter language. In the 1990s the advent of fMRI scans, PET data and the contribution of the neurobiologists brought more detailed understanding of how these electrochemical conversations, that take place between neurons, reflect the representation and coding of inner and outer experience within the mind, and the responses of the human mind to such experience. Circuits of neurons, engaged in electrochemical conversations, develop as synaptic connections are made: complex circuits form systems or networks. Some pathways are local but others are myelinated (covered in fatty white tissue) for effective conduction to distant neural structures. Increased activity in the developing brain leads to increased synaptic complexity. As the mind-brain experiences new patterns of stimuli from the outside world, new synaptic pathways are made and local biochemical and electric connections change. As each person's experience is different, so there are different patterns of connectivity in every brain-mind.

Chemicals in the brain

Neurotransmitters are chemicals that transmit messages from brain cell to brain cell, that is, from neuron to neuron. Some neurotransmitters are also neuromodulators that modify effects in the brain. Many different types of neurotransmitters have been found and some are of particular significance for the understanding of the brain-mind. *Dopamine* is involved in arousal, curiosity-interest-expectancy responses and the dreaming process, *noradrenaline* (known as *norepinephrine* in the United States) enables physical and mental arousal and heightens mood, and is involved in the brain's emergency response to trauma. *Serotonin* regulates mood, emotion and anxiety, *acetylcholine* is involved in attention, learning and memory, *glutamate* is the major excitatory chemical and enables short- and long-term memory processing, and *gamma-aminobutyric acid* (GABA) acts as a chemical guard between cells preventing over-activity that might lead to cell destruction. The group known as *endorphins* (endogenous opiates) modify traumatic experience, reduce stress, induce calm and reward bonding. Some, such as glutamate or GABA, act throughout the brain. Others, such as serotonin and dopamine, have specific pathways that enable the execution of their particular functions. For example in the case of dopamine, Carter (2000) notes that

> a stimulus from outside . . . or from the body . . . is registered by the limbic system which creates an urge which registers consciously as desire. The cortex then instructs the body to act in whatever way is necessary to achieve its desire. The activity sends messages back to the limbic system which releases opioid-like neurotransmitters which raise circulating dopamine levels and create a feeling of satisfaction.

(Carter 2000: 95)

The structure of the brain

The brain is divided into two asymmetrical halves or hemispheres (see Figure 2.2). Each hemisphere develops in a rather specialized

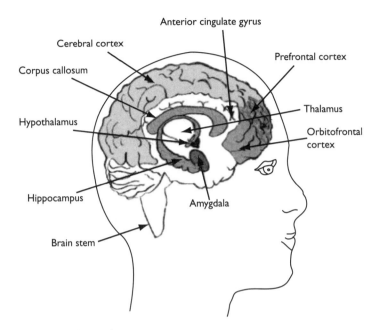

Figure 2.2 The human brain

Source: Gerhardt (2004: 35)

way, carrying out specific functions. Initially it was thought that each function was located in a very specific area, and to some extent this is true, but it is now thought that these densely connected areas, at least in some cases, may merge imperceptibly into one another rather than having very discrete edges. If either hemisphere is damaged or removed very early in life, the other half may be able to take over some of the functions that would normally be located in the other. This may also happen but only in an extremely limited way in later life, for example after physical trauma or stroke.

Although asymmetrical in shape, the two hemispheres match each other in that there tends to be two of each different module within the very complex modular system that goes to make up the internal structure of the brain, one located in each hemisphere. I will follow the convention of using the singular for each part but noting when it is thought to be more active in one hemisphere (for example the hippocampus in the left hemisphere and the amygdala in the right).

The brain may be thought of as in three parts: the brain stem (the brain's ancient core), a midbrain (which evolved later) and then (last to come on the scene) the cortex, the massively folded 'thinking-cap' that covers the brain.

The brain stem

The brain stem consists of connections to the spinal cord and thus to the whole body. The area immediately joining the spinal cord, known as the medulla oblongata, regulates bodily functions that occur beneath the level of conscious awareness such as heart and respiration rates and blood pressure. Near the top of the brain stem hangs the cerebellum, or little ancient brain that has been superseded in modern humans by the cerebral cortex.

The midbrain

The parts of the midbrain that deal with emotion and memory (including the thalamus, the hypothalamus, the amygdala and the hippocampus) are sometimes described together as the limbic system. This, however, is a theoretical concept rather than a description of a clearly identifiable area. Some regard the term as unhelpful as there is considerable disagreement as to what should be included in it. Others use it as shorthand for the part of the brain which deals with emotion and which is densely connected to the orbito-frontal cortex, the control centre in the cortex for the processing of emotion.

The cerebral cortex

Covering the other parts of the brain is the cerebrum, with its densely folded thin outer layer known as the cerebral cortex. Each hemisphere of the cerebral cortex has four separate lobes. The occipital lobe is at the back of the head and deals in the main with visual processing. Lying at the side is the temporal lobe which deals with some aspects of memory and with sound and speech comprehension (usually in the left hemisphere). Situated at the top of the head is the parietal lobe that deals mainly with movement and sensation. The powerful frontal lobes carry responsibility for executive decision-making.

The right hemisphere

There is increasing interest in the particular role of the right hemisphere of the brain in human development. It is more mature at birth than the late developing left hemisphere, therefore Schore (2002) argues that the right hemisphere has a crucial role to play in infant development (see Chapter 3 for a more detailed discussion of this). The right hemisphere processes the baby's earliest response to the stimuli that bombard it from the outside world. From birth the right brain, especially the amygdala, processes the baby's earliest experience of the primary caretaker, especially her face and the emotions reflected on it (Sieratzki and Woll 1996). By 3 months old the anterior cingulate is on line preparing the baby for experiences of socialization. Later, from 10 months onwards, the prefrontal cortex matures and enables the baby to experience a more mature kind of relating, ultimately leading to the ability to self-regulate, to deal with experience of separateness and of shame. Panksepp suggests that our right cerebral hemisphere tends to be emotionally deep and negativistic (Panksepp 2003: 10). The right amygdala processes frightening faces but its reaction may be modified by the orbitofrontal cortex, unless extreme stress has led to severe pruning of the neuronal connections that would have facilitated this (Schore 2001c). Other studies emphasize the right hemisphere's receptive involvement in the early experience of emotional prosody, that is the lilt and rhythm of the human voice (Nakamura et al. 1999). Siegel suggests self-soothing as a further function of the right hemisphere (Siegel 2003: 14).

Schore refers to a large number of studies that together establish that the early forming right hemisphere stores an internal working model of the attachment relationship that then determines the individual's characteristic strategies of affect regulation for coping and survival (Schore 2003a: 245). Schore points out its capacities for appraisal, particularly of emotion, and for the association of emotion with ideas and thought, for self-reflective awareness and for theory of mind tasks with affective components (Schore 2003a: 63). Devinsky discusses the function of the right hemisphere and concludes that it is dominant for awareness of the physical and emotional self and for a primordial sense of self (Devinsky 2000: 69). Decety and Chaminade marshal evidence to establish their view that 'the inferior parietal cortex and the prefrontal cortex in the right hemisphere play a special role in the essential ability to recognize self from others, and in the way the self represents the other' (Decety and Chaminade 2003: 577). They therefore understand the self as both special and social, and self–other interaction as the key to the development of the self. They note that 'self awareness, empathy, identification with others, and more generally intersubjective processes, are largely dependent upon right hemisphere resources, which are the first to develop' (Decety and Chaminade 2003: 596).

The left hemisphere

With the growth of the late maturing left brain, by 2–3 years old the child develops increased linguistic and analytic ability, functions that are located in this hemisphere. This enables a new experience of agency, of relating and of separateness. The development of the hippocampus enables explicit or declarative memory. Three key areas assist this development. The dorsolateral prefrontal cortex where we are able to consider our thought and feelings is the site of working memory, that is information held in mind for the needs of the immediate moment, perhaps formed from current experience or possibly reassembled from long-term memory for current use (see Chapter 4 for a detailed discussion). The other two areas are the anterior cingulate and the hippocampus, which tags time and place to memory and assists in its storage and retrieval. Together the three play a major role in the development of the social self that is able to communicate with others (Gerhardt 2004). These processes can occur effectively only if there is good interhemispheric communication. Development is sometimes impaired where there has been severe, sustained or multilayered trauma (Teicher 2000, 2002). Part of the extreme fear response associated with trauma is to inhibit the speech centres located in this side of the brain. It may be this that leads to the impairment of the corpus callosum (the major link route between the hemispheres), observed by Teicher (2002) in his large-scale studies.

A complex communication system

How to conceptualize the structure and functioning of the brain in an accessible way for the reader has exercised my mind and those of many writers before me. Some have resorted to metaphor, for example the orchestra (Goldberg 2001) and the landscape (Carter

2000), others choose to use the language of computer science or of architecture. Nothing seems to describe adequately this amazing living entity, that is itself part of a living organism. It is the control centre of the mind-brain-body being and yet contains within itself a further control centre, the prefrontal cortex. The human brain has evolved over the millennia in response to environmental challenge, and latterly to the challenge of the development of language. It is unique in each individual, not only formed in that individual in response to inherited predispositions, but also very much shaped by the environment in which the individual develops. It develops most particularly in response to the experience of relationship, especially with the primary care-giver. The development of the brain and the brain-mind is fundamentally associative and relational. Each brain develops as a result of its interaction with that which is felt inwardly in the body and that which affects the person from outside that is, in the first instance, the primary care-giver. Its plasticity, that is its capacity for change, is at its height in the first three years of life and again in adolescence. This plasticity continues throughout the lifespan.

For the moment I will try to pursue the metaphor of a complex communication system, such as may be represented on a road or rail map. If you look at either the road or rail systems of most countries, one thing is immediately apparent: virtually all the major routes radiate from/to the capital, which is in effect the control centre.

The control centre

The prefrontal cortex

Much the same may be said of the prefrontal cortex, the executive control centre of the brain, located in the cortex, the 'thinking-cap' of the brain (which is the latest part of the brain to develop in evolutionary terms and which is most highly developed in humans). It has direct connections to virtually every part of the brain. The ventromedial or orbitofrontal part of this (the middle part, behind the orbit of the eyes) is unique because it is so close to all three major regions of the brain. 'Its central location anatomically enables it to integrate the cortex, limbic structure and brain stem into a functional whole' (Siegel 2003: 21).

The prefrontal cortex acts as the emotional executive of the right brain as it has strong neural connections into the emotional systems located in the early developing right hemisphere that is dominant in the earliest years, until the late developing left brain is able to come on line. The integration made possible by the activity of this part of the brain may be the means by which self-regulation is achieved. Schore (2003a) comments that

> attachment experiences, face to face transactions of affect synchrony between care-giver and infant, directly influence the imprinting, the circuit wiring of the orbitofrontal cortex ... known to begin a major maturational change at 10–12 months and to complete a critical period of growth in the middle to the end of the second year.
>
> (Schore 2003a: 60)

Gerhardt (2004) cites Chugani's study which demonstrated that Romanian orphans 'cut off from close bonds with an adult by being left in their cots all day, unable to make relationships, had a virtual black hole where their orbitofrontal cortex should be' (Chugani et al. 2001, cited in Gerhardt 2004: 38).

The communication systems

Edelman and Tononi (2000: 42–50) identify several communication systems in the brain that are vital for its effective functioning and for the achieving of consciousness (Figure 2.3).

> (A) The top diagram shows the thalamocortical system – a dense meshwork of reentrant connectivity between the thalamus and the cortex and between different cortical regions through so-called corticocortical fibers. (B) The middle diagram depicts long, polysynaptic loops that are arranged in parallel and that leave the cortex, enter the so-called cortical appendages (indicated here are the basal ganglia and the cerebellum), and return to the cortex. (C) The bottom diagram indicates one of the diffusely projecting value systems (the noradrenergic locus coeruleus), which distributes a 'hairnet' of fibers all over the brain and can release the neuromodulator noradrenaline.
>
> (Edelman and Tononi 2000: 43)

The dense network

The dense network is comprised of the thalamocortical system with hundreds of specialized areas, each containing tens of thousands of

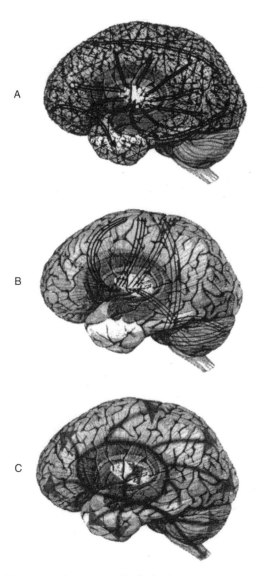

Figure 2.3 Communications systems in the brain

Source: Edelman and Tononi (2000: 43)

neuronal groups. All these neuronal groups are linked by convergent or divergent, reciprocally organized connections that go to make up a single tight mesh.

The long loops systems

The long loops systems make up the routes that link the cortex to and from a set of its appendages, the cerebellum, the basal ganglia (which includes the amygdala) and the hippocampus. Each route forms a separate loop, specialized to carry out its own unique set of tasks.

The fan-like systems

The fan-like systems form pathways for the hormonal systems (noradrenergic, serotinergic, dopaminergic, cholinergic and histaminergic). Edelman and Tononi (2000) note that the firing of neurons in each of these systems releases its neuromodulator and note that these powerful hormones are capable of affecting not only neural activity but also neural plasticity enabling adaptive change within the brain-mind-body.

The major inter-hemisphere link routes

The most significant inter-hemisphere link route is formed by the corpus callosum, a curved white band of tissue that connects the two hemispheres, consisting of approximately 200 million nerve fibres and acting as the main route of communication between the right and left hemispheres. It enables continuous exchange of information between the two hemispheres of the brain. The anterior commisure connects the limbic system in each of the two hemispheres enabling exchange of emotional information at an unconscious level.

The information systems

The thalamus, hypothalamus and basal ganglia

Together these three subcortical structures in the midbrain are responsible for perception 'outside', via the senses (thalamus), 'inside', inner visceral states (the hypothalamus) and action (basal ganglia, including the amygdala). The thalamus is able to process sensory information from outside the body arriving from the different brain areas involved in initial reception of such information. It is closely linked to the hypothalamus that monitors information from inside the body. The hypothalamus is a vital endocrine centre. The hormones it secretes enable neural processes to work associatively throughout the brain and body.

The amygdala

The amygdala, a tiny area at the heart of the limbic system, is thought to be especially important in the processing of emotion in the right brain and is responsible for the emergency response system of the brain. In the face of perceived threat, it operates pre-cognitively to organize an immediate and total brain-body response. At the same time it informs the cortex where a more measured view may be taken, the immediate threat already being responded to by the instant processes activated by the amygdala. Implicit, unconscious, emotional 'memories' of earliest experiences are also stored there. They form the early patterning that dictates the most deeply held ways of being and behaving that become part of our emotional repertoire for the rest of our lives. Within this store are implicit memory patterns of previous traumatic experience which inform the amygdala's response at moments of crisis. It is over-reaction of this system that gives rise to the symptoms that manifest themselves in post-traumatic stress disorder (PTSD). LeDoux stresses that the amygdala 'is a critical site of learning because of its central location between input and output stations' (LeDoux 1999: 114).

The hippocampus

The hippocampus is associated with activity in the left hemisphere and tags time and place to memory and is responsible for the encoding of long-term memory.

The brain stem core

From the brain stem core at the base of the brain many pathways arise, reaching to even the distant parts of the brain, ensuring their activation. Some routes from the brain stem are biochemically specific, involving a particular neurotransmitter, others are biochemically complex and involve several neurotransmitters (Goldberg 2001: 29). The nerves of the brain stem extend from the spinal cord and therefore form the brain-body link route.

Governing principles of the brain-mind

The network development of the brain-mind depends on progression from simplicity to complexity, via patterning

The brain's modification of synaptic connections comes about through its response to its interaction with both the inner and outer world. The total environment includes that which impinges from outside, often in the form of the experience that arises out of significant relationships, and that which is experienced from within as the body feeds information about bodily states of being. Mind responds to the changes that occur in the brain as a result of experience; brain is therefore modified again in response to mind. Plasticity allows the possibility of this continual modification of earlier 'patterning' that has become established in the brain, based on earlier experience. Schank (1999) notes that such modification occurs when the brain experiences expectation failures. Thus the brain is able to learn from experience and to modify future expectation in the light of it. Much of the exchange between analyst and patient relies on this aspect of the mind-brain relationship. Networks within the brain connect in a multiplicity of ways, permitting the most complex patterns of information processing. These neural activity patterns provide the elements of which meaning is made (Freeman 1999). Cozolino (2002) points out that

> Transcortical networks in both hemispheres feed highly processed sensory-motor information forward to the frontal cortex. Simultaneously, multiple hierarchical networks, which loop up and down through the cortex, limbic system and brainstem, provide the frontal cortex with visceral, behavioural and emotional information.
>
> (Cozolino 2002: 132)

Networks provide the circuitry of emotion linking the amygdala and anterior cingulate to the orbitofrontal cortex that is the senior executive of the emotional brain. Other networks provide the prefrontal cortex with information from the senses and the body. Neural pathways enable integration of the hippocampal memory system, which tags time and place to explicit memory, with the amygdaloidal memory system, which retains emotional and somatic experience in implicit memory. As these regions are biased towards the left and right hemispheres respectively integration is enhanced across the top–down and left–right axes of information processing (Cozolino 2002: 140). Our knowledge of the complex circuits that form systems with a specific function, such as fear, rage or lust, has become clearer because of the work of those who study affective neuroscience.

As the data that comes to each individual in each moment is in a sense unique, the patterns that build are also unique to each individual. The unique patterns of connectivity in each brain give birth to its unique mind. Freeman comments: 'the dynamics that isolates the meaning in each brain from all others, endowing each person with ultimate privacy, and loneliness as well . . . creates the challenge of creating companionship with others through communication' (Freeman 1999: 12). The global patterns of awareness developing in each hemisphere, arising from the integration of component subsystems and experienced as a sequence may be a way of describing consciousness. Any view of consciousness must extend beyond the brain to include the body, and beyond a purely neural explanation to include the effects of interactions with the environment; only thus can self-awareness be fully understood (Horgan 1999: 299). Horgan's (1999) article provides an excellent summary of the varied positions currently held in the scientific world on the vexing puzzle of consciousness.

Mirroring the other

Considerable research both in humans and animals has led to the conclusion that much of human development occurs by means of a mirroring process. The phrase 'monkey see, monkey do' has come to describe a process whereby similar brain activity is apparent in both the brain of a monkey that performs a motor action i.e. reaching for and eating a banana, and in the brain of the monkey who observes that action. These results were derived from the research of Gallese, Fadiga, Fogassi and Rizzolatti (2002) and Rizzolatti, Fadiga, Fogassi and Gallese (1999). Decety and Chaminade (2003) observe that transcranial magnetic stimulation (TMS) and EEG techniques have been used to demonstrate similar effects in humans. They conclude that 'action observation involves neural regions similar to those engaged during actual action production' and go on to establish a basis for neural empathy by arguing that 'perception of emotion activates the neural mechanisms responsible for the generation of emotions' (Decety and Chaminade 2003: 583–4). They conclude that understanding that others are like us, at the psychological level, develops as one represents the mental activities and processes of others by generating similar activities and processes in oneself (Decety and Chaminade 2003: 582). What is so striking about this for therapists and analysts is that it provides a sound neuroscientific basis for the transference/countertransference process and establishes an indissoluble link between those processes and the earliest development of mind.

Association areas

Certain areas of the brain have key functions in coordinating information and response to that information. The amygdala assesses external danger and initiates necessary response from the body as well as passing the relevant information to the higher cortical areas of the brain. The anterior cingulate brings together sensory, autonomic and emotional information and passes it to the orbital area of the prefrontal cortex that organizes emotional experience and affect regulation. The temporal lobes also bring together information from the senses and integrate it with emotional and bodily information received from the amygdala, particularly concerning fear (Cozolino 2002). The prefrontal cortex is becoming increasingly recognized as playing a key role in self-consciousness, self-ownership, self-agency and self-other representations. Re-entry is a notable feature of the human brain. Edelman and Tononi define it as 'the on-going, recursive interchange of parallel signals between reciprocally connected areas of the brain' (Edelman and Tononi 2000: 48). It is the process by which information is shared between different areas of the brain and that makes possible the synchronization and coordination of the mutual activities of the different areas.

Plasticity and connectivity

Plasticity enables the change and learning that occurs in analysis. Although the plasticity of the brain enables this learning to continue throughout the life cycle, in adulthood the development of new neurons is uncertain. However, the development of new neural pathways is commonplace as synapses change every time we record an experience. Canli (2004: 1118) cites a number of studies that demonstrate that 'the connectivity between different brain regions can vary as a function of attention'. It is here that the often intense engagement of analyst and analysand, resulting from the transference, becomes crucial. He also emphasizes the related concept of 'neural connectivity [that is that] the role that one region plays in neural representation of a psychological function depends on the activity in other regions at the same time' (Canli 2004: 1119). More brain centres light up in response to metaphor than any other form of human communication, thus indicating the formation of new neural pathways (Levin 1997 and Modell 1997, cited in Pally 2000: 132). Lakoff and Johnson (1999) argue that it is early bodily experience, particularly that of movement from which metaphor arises. They describe as primary metaphor that which arises out of bodily experience in early childhood and secondary metaphor as that which develops from primary metaphor, or from common knowledge, or widely held cultural beliefs. Ekstrom cites 'affection is warmth' as an example of primary metaphor arising from the primary experience of 'feeling warm while being held affectionately' (Ekstrom 2004: 667). The importance of working with metaphor as a way of utilizing the brain's plasticity underpins the clinical approach advocated in this book. It will be manifest in the transference, in dreams and the mirroring of the early dyad in the experience of the analytic dyad as they work together. New neural connections are not created as entirely new entities but rather are added to pre-existing connections; analytic work painstakingly builds on experience from session to session in just this way. The pithy phrase 'cells that fire together wire together' is often used to describe this process. Mark Solms, in debate with Susan Greenfield (at the Institute of Psychoanalysis, London, October 2002), suggested that the difference between conscious and unconscious might indicate the degree of connectivity established.

Brain-body links

The release of hormones and the reaction of the skeletal muscles mean that brain activity engenders body changes in what may truly be thought of as the mind-brain-body being. 'The body is the theatre (McDougall 1989), the body speaks (Sidoli 2000), the body remembers (Rothschild 2000) and the body keeps the score (van der Kolk 1996)' see (Wilkinson 2003: 242). The mirroring response is one important aspect of brain-body linking. Buccino et al. (2001, cited in Decety and Chaminade 2003) have shown that watching another's action (the 'monkey see, monkey do' principle at work, that is the mirroring of the neural pathways involving a specific motor action described earlier) activates the premotor cortex in a somatotopical manner, for example watching actions involving hand, mouth or foot activates their respective representations in the watcher's brain, then that empathic, imitative, imaginative 'body' experience becomes 'knowable' in mind. Heilman et al. (1998, cited in Decety and Chaminade 2003) in their discussion of brain-body links suggest that representation of the body in the brain-mind is continuously updated by feedback in both directions.

Experience inevitably comes to us through our senses, feelings are rooted in bodily experience of emotion or affect. We speak of 'going red with rage' (increased blood supply as the result of the fight response of the sympathetic nervous system), we may then go on to say, 'I froze with fright, the sound brought a chill to my heart' (the onset of the response parasympathetic nervous system, setting in motion the shutdown or freeze state that comes into operation in the face of the realization of overwhelming experience). These systems are discussed more fully in Chapter 5. Experiencing sadness, we might describe it by saying that 'my eyes filled with tears', or its opposite might be described as 'my heart was filled with joy'. In the face of trauma, hippocampal shutdown may mean that the body is the only place in which the nature of the traumatic experience is 'remembered' (van der Kolk 1996; Rothschild 2000). It is the body that will teach the observant therapist how to work with the trauma.

In the consulting-room

One speculates that in the consulting-room through the revisiting of experiences that went to establish attachment in the first year of life, new neural pathways and patterns of connectivity in the right hemisphere of the brain may be established. Communication between the hemispheres means that experience can then be put into words and processed by the left. Solomon has described this kind of development as 'eye-talk that leads to "I" talk'

(H.M. Solomon, unpublished communication, 1999). Left–right integration enables the patient to put feelings into words, to think about feelings, to experience and name feelings in the mind rather than experiencing them in the body. Research suggests that 'restoring neural integration requires the simultaneous re-regulation of networks on both vertical and horizontal planes' (Cozolino 2002: 30). For example, as in the material given from Harriet (see Chapter 4), Xanthe and Susan (Chapter 8) and Mark (Chapter 9), a dream, a vivid, visual, emotional, right cerebral experience becomes available to the left hemisphere, dominant for language, through the analytic process, which is itself made possible by such containment. It is the interactive experience within the analytic dyad that enables the development of regulatory capacity and reflective function.

Conversely care must be taken to avoid a situation where patients may unconsciously seek retraumatization in the consulting-room in order to experience an endorphin 'high' to which they have become accustomed in early and repetitive experiences of trauma. Scaer (2001a) observes that 'children abused by their care-giver will experience increased levels of endorphins as part of the traumatization and freeze response' and that such children 'will also be rewarded by the presence of the increased endorphin levels associated with reattachment and bonding to the abuser' (Scaer 2001a: 88). Scaer also points out the parallel pattern that occurs with female spousal abuse.

Patients who have experienced such patterns of opiate reward will present in the consulting-room also unconsciously seeking endorphinergic reward. Thus they may continually seek to re-experience trauma in what may be thought of as an addictive state of mind. Such a pattern may also occur when a patient attaches to a therapist who unconsciously works in an abusive way, or is experienced as doing so in the transference. In each situation the patient unconsciously seeks the endorphinergic effects, with ensuing opiate reward, of the abusive situation. Re-experiencing or re-enactment in the consulting-room of this kind will become addictive rather than therapeutic. Thus the therapist must consider carefully the appropriateness of any re-experiencing or re-enactment that occurs in the consulting-room. This is discussed more fully and illustrated with clinical examples in Chapter 5.

Conclusion

The mind-brain-body being that is the human being develops associatively. In health and in trauma the brain and body are intimately and inevitably involved in the building of that which becomes represented in mind. The dissociative response to trauma may represent a breaking of those links, in order to avoid psychic pain. Thus mind that is fundamentally associative becomes dissociative as a defensive measure, leaving trauma to be expressed as it was experienced, that is in the body. Stress hormones affect the whole body, thus brain changes engender body changes. Cortisol levels are elevated initially and this is particularly damaging in children where stress is sustained over time. 'Unusually high levels of cortisol levels from constant stress slow physical growth, delay sexual maturity and can slow the growth of brain cells' (M. Davies 2002: 428). However, the long-term effects of trauma result in lowered cortisol levels with concurrent adverse effects on the immune system (Yehuda 1998: 97). Dealing with the level of anxiety in the body, that is maintaining a dissociative state in order to avoid the unbearable psychic pain that a more associated way of being would bring, consumes considerable energy with significant psychological and biological consequences to the person concerned (Rosen and Schulkin 1998). Increased levels of energy and creativity may be dramatic in patients whose analyses successfully address trauma-related anxiety. Sound therapy requires an understanding of mind, brain and body. Now such knowledge is available, nothing less will do.

Chapter 3

The early development of the brain-mind

One can actually see the conscious mind coming into existence.
(Jung 1954d: para. 103)

Early mind: associative, relational and implicit

The thread that runs through this book is one of coming into mind as a developmental achievement which in good enough circumstances unfolds associatively in relation to the primary care-giver. As the right brain develops early, it is a key player in early developmental achievement, storing early internal models of being and relating deep in implicit, amygdaloidal, emotional memory. The sparsity of connections in the infant brain (see Figure 3.1) means that the child is much like a book waiting to be written, to a certain extent the content is already determined, but the form and the emphases that will emerge are as yet unknown. The individual's brain and mind will owe a huge amount to the infant's and growing child's experiences of nurture, with mother, with father and with significant others.

But is it a case of nature (our genes) or nurture (environmental stimulus) or both?

The psyche of the child in its preconscious state is anything but a *tabula rasa*: it is already preformed in a recognisably individual way, and is moreover equipped with all specifically human instincts, as well as with the *a priori* foundations of the higher functions. On this complicated base the ego arises.
(Jung 1962: 381–2)

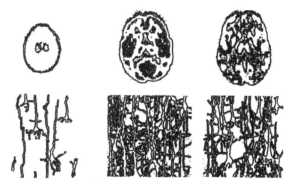

Neural connections are sparse at birth (left), but new connections are made at a terrific rate during infancy and by the age of 6 (middle) they are at maximum density. Thereafter they decrease again as unwanted connections die back (right). Adults can increase neural connections throughout their life by learning new things. But if the brain is not used, the connections will become further depleted.

Figure 3.1 The development of neural connections in the developing brain

Source: Carter (2000: 18)

In this, Jung anticipated the insights of neurologists, such as Damasio, who comments:

> The brain does not begin its day as a *tabula rasa*. The brain is imbued at the start of life with knowledge regarding how the organism should be managed . . . the brain brings along innate knowledge and automated know-how, predetermining many ideas of the body.
>
> (Damasio 2004: 205)

But just what is hard-wired? Decety and Chaminade (2003), in a ground-breaking article, make clear, once and for all, that current research has set on one side the older notion of 'infants as social isolates, devoid of any intersubjective link between self and other, or being in a state where they confuse the self and the other' (Decety and Chaminade 2003: 577). They marshal a considerable amount of scientific evidence, some from recent neuro-imaging studies, to show that newborns can distinguish between their own touch and the touch of another (Rochat and Hespos 1997), that neonates imitate facial gestures of another and can do so at less than 1 hour old (Meltzoff and Moore 1995) and that understanding another person is initially a form of embodied experience (Gallagher and

Meltzoff 1996). By 15 months old children imitate the things they can understand (Mandler and McDonough 2000). Very young infants can distinguish between non-humans and humans and preferentially attribute mental states to the humans (Johnson 2000). By 18 months old children imitate the actions of humans but not of objects (Legerstee 1991; Meltzoff 1995). Decety and Chaminade (2003) cite a considerable amount of evidence, of which I have tried to give a flavour, which leads them to conclude that 'these studies establish that human infants are motivated for social interaction and suggest that the development of an awareness of other minds is rooted in the implicit notion that others are like the self' (Decety and Chaminade 2003: 580). They conclude that there is good evidence that reciprocal imitation plays a vital part in the early development of the implicit self (Rochat 1999, cited in Decety and Chaminade 2003). As the self is fundamentally associative and its development based on psychological identification, mechanisms such as transference and countertransference are rooted in the very earliest experience of mind. They mirror processes which are early, implicit and emotional. The emotional power of such processes may take some by surprise but how could it be otherwise, considering their rootedness in early right brain experience, the more so when that experience has been traumatic?

Although the brain is hard-wired in this way from the beginning the development of mind is thus very much dependent on each individual's experience of relating to others, the initial development of mind arising from intimate interactions with the mother and also the father. Thus the part played by genes has to be acknowledged but its limitations also understood. Canli (2004: 1121, citing Hamer 2002) explains that a genetic understanding of human behaviour is 'oversimplified if it relies on a direct linear relationship between genes and behaviour . . . rather . . . one needs to incorporate the brain, the environment, and gene expression networks in future models'. Caspi et al. (2003) stress the importance of the interaction of genes and environment in shaping the human response. LeDoux (2002) emphasizes that genes only shape the broad outline of mental and behavioural functions, that inheritance may bias us in certain directions, but that many environmental factors, most particularly the primary care-giver, affect how one's genes are expressed. He concludes that nature and nurture are just different ways of wiring synapses in the brain (LeDoux 2002). Jungians, such as Knox, writing from an interactionist, developmental viewpoint have already begun to explore the significance of this for our understanding of archetypal theory (Knox 2003).

Relational development of mind

From the beginning then, the development of mind is dependent on experience of relating to others, the initial development of mind arising from intimate interactions with the mother and also the father. Knox comments that 'mind and meaning emerge out of developmental processes and the experience of interpersonal relationships rather than existing *a priori*' (Knox 2004: 16). Earliest experiences of emotional states arise out of bodily experiences in relation to the primary care-giver. Panksepp, Schore and many others emphasize an experience-dependent understanding of the development of the self from an inner core self. They stress the relational, intersubjective nature of the development of the individual self. Thus we may think of the individual as a mind-brain-body being that has emerged from the experience of the earliest and most fundamental experiences of relating. Both nature and nurture have had a part to play in the growth and development of the neuronal connections that go to make up the individual mind. Siegel comments: 'Relationships may not only be encoded in memory but may also shape the very circuits that enable memory to be processed and self-regulation to be achieved' (Siegel 2003: 14).

A Jungian developmental view

Jung stressed the profound effects of the early experiences in life. Fordham (1976), drawing on the work of Stein (1967), understood that 'the self has defence systems designed to preserve individual identity and establish and maintain the difference between self and not-self' (Fordham 1976: 90). Fordham described the healthy processes of deintegration and integration by which the infant begins to develop a sense of self in the world, which we have seen exemplified in Jacques. Astor (1998) comments: 'Important in this process was the mother's capacity to receive and make sense of the baby's communication in such a way that the baby took in from its mother's attention . . . that it . . . could be understood' (Astor 1998: 12). Fordham emphasized that, when the infant self is threatened by overwhelming experiences it cannot process, the threat of disintegration occurs and the infant self protects itself by a retreat from the world into an autistic state (Fordham 1976: 88–93). Solomon (1998) emphasized that

> when early trauma has taught a young self that searching for experiences that could lead to growth and relation to another is ... psychologically dangerous, leaving the self open to damage and exploitation, the self has no other recourse but to withdraw back into itself.
>
> (Solomon 1998: 236)

Fordham argued that 'if a baby is subjected to noxious stimuli of a pathogenic nature ... a persistent over-reaction of the defence system may start to take place' (Fordham 1976: 91). I now understand such a process as the defensive development of neural pathways in order to protect the self, that is fundamentally associative and relational, but which is driven into a protective way of being by adverse environmental experience, usually in the relation with the primary care-giver.

Ellen

Ellen, a 7-year-old girl who had been severely abused by her parents, had just moved into foster care and begun twice-weekly psychotherapy with a child psychotherapist. In her therapy she used metaphorical play to explore her pain. In an early session she corralled the toy wild animals in a 'nasty prison pen'. She explained that they longed to jump free to get to a nice house that was quite near but they could not jump. Instead they crept cautiously and warily right around the edge of the room, clinging to the skirting board. As she played, the child battered the therapist with words non-stop to avoid the possibility of any penetrative speech entering her. The therapist felt it was all absolutely unbearable. She managed to interpret something of her countertransference, speaking first of the plight of the animals and then how the child might be feeling. There was an internal shift from a feeling of utter helplessness to the use of an omnipotent defence. The safe words had brought change and the child used what she called 'magic' to omnipotently enable the last animals to jump freely to a safe place (C.V. Hart, unpublished communication, 2002).

Early development

The immature brain at birth has uncommitted, immature connections, built in the main from the inside. A newborn baby's senses are flooded with the many sights, sounds, smells, tastes and textures from the outside world as well as those sensations and feelings that arise from within. As the baby's brain responds by growing more neuronal connections than will ultimately be needed, a neural pruning then takes place as cells without inputs die, 'the use it or lose it' principle at work. Schore reports that an MRI scan study on infants shows that the volume of the brain increases rapidly during the first 2 years, that infants under 2 years of age show higher right than left volume, that the normal adult appearance is seen at 2 years and that all major fibre tracts can be identified by 3 years of age (Schore 2003a: 237).

Early attachment

In 'good enough' circumstances in infancy, secure attachment is established over the first year of life, through the holding and smiling and vocal exchanges of the first months of life, and what Schore describes as multimodal high intensity positive affect exchanges of the second 6 months of life, by which the mother imprints the infant's postnatally developing nervous system. Schore explains that this very rapid form of learning 'irreversibly stamps early experience upon the developing nervous system and mediates attachment bond formation' (Schore 2003a: 277). Thus mind is made by the healthy interaction with another mind, that of the primary care-giver.

Patterns in the mind

Schore describes the mother's face as 'the most potent visual stimulus in the child's world' (Schore 2002: 18). Gerhardt describes the effects of the mother's smile on the baby's developing system:

> his own nervous system becomes pleasurably aroused and his own heart rate goes up. These processes trigger off a biochemical response ... a pleasure neuropeptide called beta-endorphin is released into circulation and specifically into the orbitofrontal region of the brain.
>
> (Gerhardt 2004: 41)

We've explored something of this in the extracts from Jacques' early experience described in Chapter 1. As a baby experiences consistently warm empathic exchanges with his mother, over time, patterns of expectation begin to build in the baby's brain, being held brings a sense of warmth and the beginnings of an awareness of good feelings arising from intimate contact with another. These patterns that build in the baby's brain-mind, stored in implicit or emotional memory, and affecting the way the baby begins to expect encounters with another to be, have been variously described. Gerhardt summarizes:

> Daniel Stern (1985) calls them representations of interactions that have been generalized (RIGS). John Bowlby called them 'internal working models' (1969). Wilma Bucci calls them 'emotional schemas (1997). Robert Clyman calls them 'procedural memory' (1991).
>
> (Gerhardt 2004: 24)

The interactions that occur between mothers and babies have been closely studied and basic types of attachment have been identified, these patterns of attachment become long-lasting and are recognizable in adult patients in the consulting-room. Through the transference/countertransference experience the therapist can become aware of the nature of the patient's earliest attachment pattern. Understanding that pattern will be crucial for effective work to occur at a relational level.

Patterns of attachment

In good enough circumstances the mother–baby dyad is able to establish a warm, empathic way of being together which results in a secure attachment, one from which the growing child will step confidently into the wider world. But sadly in less propitious circumstances, an infant may see alarm, fear or terror on the mother's face and the baby's face and feelings will come to mirror those of the mother. Schore explains that in the mother–infant exchanges that occur between such dyads the baby mirrors 'the rhythmic structures of the mother's dysregulated states, and ... this synchronization is registered in the firing patterns of the stress-sensitive corticolimbic regions of the infant's brain that are in a critical period of growth' (Schore 2003a: 251).

Schore notes that the image of the mother's face directly stimulates the dopaminergic and noradrenergic pathways, that are thought to be associated with anticipation, in this case of terror, of the orbitofrontal cortex of the baby's brain.

When the baby is hungry, or wet, or sad, or uncomfortable, in good enough circumstances the state of arousal that this produces is attended to by the mother and the baby returns to a resting state. Where the mother is depressed or withdrawn she may not respond and the baby's state of distress will escalate. Where the mother responds but in a fearful, angry, terrifying or inconsistent, unpredictable way then the baby will be affected throughout the whole brain-body being. As they grow up toddlers may develop one of three identifiable responses. If they could speak about how they feel, this is what they might deep down long to say:

- the avoidant: 'I must avoid Mum's anger by avoiding a knowledge of my own difficult feelings, pushing them down, switching them off'
- the ambivalent: 'Sometimes Mum's OK, sometimes not, I must watch carefully and modify my mood and feelings to hers' (some of these children become distant and avoid others, some become anxious and clingy in their efforts to solve their dilemma)
- the disorganized: 'Mum is so unpredictable I just don't know what to do for the best, I'm afraid all the time'.

The last group will find it most difficult to manage as they seek to grow up and to relate to others in their wider world. Holmes suggests that 'in average populations about one-fifth of children are avoidant, one-sixth ambivalent, and one in twenty disorganized' in their attachment style (Holmes 1996: 7–8).

Traumatic patterns of attachment

Schore (2002) stresses that as the limbic system myelinates in the first 18 months of life at the time when the right hemisphere is in a growth spurt and before the left hemisphere has come on line so attachment experiences inevitably affect the limbic and cortical areas of the developing right hemisphere. He reminds us that when trauma (with its associated fight, flight and freeze responses) has been experienced in the context of the earliest attachment relationship then it becomes 'burned into the developing limbic and autonomic systems of the early maturing right brain, [it becomes] part of implicit memory, and [leads to] enduring structural changes that produce inefficient stress-coping mechanisms' (Schore 2002: 9).

A baby allowed to reach a state of frantic distress will, if it remains unresolved, switch off, staring into space with a glazed look. Schore (2005) suggests that if the baby continually experiences states of unbearable fear-terror or aggression emanating from the mother's face, then dissociation will become the primary regulatory process that will be resorted to throughout the lifespan. He concludes that attachment trauma 'induces an enduring impairment of . . . the primordial central integrating structure of the nascent self' (Schore 2005: ch. 9). Chefetz comments that dissociation aims to protect the self yet in its attempts to triumph over the self it actually injures the self and leads to enduring changes in subjectivity (Chefetz 2005).

Parent–infant psychotherapy

A relatively young field, arising out of a combination of analytic thought, infant observation and infancy research, trauma theory and affective neuroscience, parent–infant psychotherapy is perhaps the most important and most hopeful of all the endeavours in the field of dynamic psychotherapy.

Judith Woodhead, a Jungian analyst, works as a member of a team that has developed the Parent–Infant Project at the Anna Freud Centre, London. I wish to explore a little of the work that occurred between her and a mother–baby dyad, Anna and Nadia, described by her in a most sensitive and fascinating paper (Woodhead 2004), as a way of elucidating the underpinning that neuroscience provides for the understanding of this delicate and vital work. Woodhead makes clear that Anna and 4-month-old Nadia needed support to be able to build affective experience together so that Nadia could experience herself in a hopeful, enjoyable way in her mother's mind. Commenting on their first session together, Woodhead describes how the baby is put down to sit alone in a car seat which the mother has turned away from her and then recounts how baby and therapist experience the weight of Anna's suffering, of traumatic affect, as they both

hear the mother's torrent of words, telling of her escape from war, of terrible experiences . . . of becoming ill after her baby's birth, of emergency hospitalisations and separations from her infant during the first month of her life.

(Woodhead 2004: 147)

Drawing upon insights from affective neuroscience, Woodhead understands that 'attachment experiences are encoded and stored separately from autobiographical memories' (Woodhead 2004: 145) in the implicit (emotional) memory system, that therefore change needs to occur for the mother–infant dyad in the area of 'implicit relational knowing' and that the presence of the therapist, working in a sensitive, empathic, relational way, can help to effect this (Woodhead 2004: 145). She appreciates the urgency of intervention because of the knowledge brought to her from research that emerged during the 'decade of the brain [that indicates] that traumatic experience may impact on the size of the regions of the infant's brain and on its capacity to regulate emotion' (Woodhead 2004: 146). She is able to describe in detail the steps by which Anna, sensing the beginning of the meeting of her own needs for support and aided by an internalization of the 'mothering' attitude modelled by the therapist, becomes available to intuit her baby's needs more accurately, to begin to be able to follow her baby's clues and meet her needs more empathically, thus permitting her baby to experience the kind of support 'that permits the infant to achieve a more complex level of brain organisation' (Tronick 1998: 295, cited in Woodhead 2004: 146). We will let the trio have the last word on the subject with material from towards the end of that first session together:

> Her mother follows her intently, synchronized with her movement, unlike earlier in the session. They nuzzle their mouths together. The baby takes a strand of her mother's hair and fingers it . . . The mother says looking directly into her face, her own face lighting up, 'Waaah, what a beautiful girl'. [Woodhead comments] Anna was freed to feel . . . that she had a beautiful daughter with whom she could be in love, while Nadia could in those moments find herself, a beautiful little person, in her mother's mind.
>
> (Woodhead 2004: 155)

Socialization

Socialization experiences in the second year of life play a vital role in the maturation of the orbitofrontal regions that takes place in the second year. At about 12 months the mother begins to inhibit the child by the introduction of the word 'No'. Schore (1994) points out that it is by around 18 months old that the parasympathetic nervous system has come on line, enabling the decrease in arousal and excitement that leads to socialization. This is achieved via 'the socialisation stress induced experience dependent structural trans-forming (rewiring) of the orbitofrontal cortex' (Schore 1994: 343). It is this that enables the development of the 'braking mechanism of shame' (Schore 1994: 343).

Just as the earliest experiences are built out of 'mirroring' experiences with the primary care-giver so the earliest experiences of being part of a group, whether the wider family, the playgroup, or with toddler friends may well involve 'mirror' experiencing. Decety and Chaminade (2003) comment that 'shared representa-tions at the cortical level have been found in action, pain processing, and emotion recognition, which would give us a neurophysiological basis for the operation of social cognition' (Decety and Chaminade 2003: 584). They go on to argue that shared representations may be common to individuals within a cultural group and would be medi-ated by similar neural networks in their respective brains. Here there would seem to be room for the neural substrate of Jung's concept of the collective unconscious and of the shared 'archetypal' images that arise from it.

Finding father

It is about this time that the toddler develops a new attachment, attachment to the father who increasingly acts as a bridge to the outside world. Schore points out that a good enough attachment between father and child will function as 'an interactive regulator of fear and aggression, thereby providing a growth facilitating environment' (Schore 2003a: 287) in which the regulatory system may mature. Paternal absence and neglect at this stage may lead to lifelong 'father thirst (Abelin 1971) [or] father hunger (Herzog 1980)' (Schore 2003a: 287), and may lead to experiences where it becomes difficult for a child to separate from the mother, as there is a lack of oedipal experience that will permit the symbolic understanding necessary for this next developmental step (Wilkinson 2001; Woodhead 2004). Modell (1999) notes the devastating consequences that arise if a mother is 'unable to recognise that her child had an inner life that was separate and distinct from her own'; he says that 'recognising the uniqueness of children's inner life is equivalent to recognising they are psychically alive. It is as if their mothers failed to recognise their humanity' (Modell 1999: 77).

Mark

Mark (whose material is also included in Chapter 9 of this book) and his mother tried to maintain an idealized state of fusion; separateness was not to be conceived of; even in sleep he should be at one with his mother. Each night at bedtime she exhorted him that they should dream of each other and dream the same dream. His tongue came to express something of the quality of their relationship. His stutter appears to have acted as a barrier to protect the self from being overwhelmed by the mother. At the same time it protected him and his mother from knowing about his hatred and guilt. If only he could have spoken easily what might he have said to a mother such as his? Mark described this experience to me as that of 'being in one skin with his mother' (Wilkinson 2001: 268). Affeld-Niemeyer describes the loss of instinctual experience and reality sense in such patients as 'an extreme regression to a primary undifferentiated stage of development: that of "ambiguity" and "identity"' (Affeld-Niemeyer 1995: 37–8). I saw Mark, who presented with complaints about his stutter, for ten years and for most of that time he attended four times a week. In the early stages of the analysis when he stuttered in the consulting-room it was with a soft, gentle prolongation of certain sounds, reminiscent of early lalling. He had most difficulty with 'm' as he sought to say 'mother'; my name became Ma . . . Ma . . . Margaret. This contrasted strongly with the later phases of the analysis when he became more aware of a different kind of mothering from the analyst-mother, which made possible the beginnings of experience of separateness and some awareness of his feelings of hate. Usually Mark seemed to be trying to control an explosion of anger and to be coming closer to an awareness of his underlying hatred of his controlling mother, then his stutter would intensify and while it remained relatively soft the words that caused difficulty changed; in one such session he had prolonged difficulty with both 'battle' and 'bite' (Wilkinson 2001).

The development of language would appear to be an intrinsic part of the process of separating from mother, that is taking language from your mother, using it in your own way and being allowed to do so. The need for language implies separateness, and the use of language acknowledges the separateness and the need to communicate across the space between self and mother. Hand in hand with that realization comes the need to 'name' mother and to 'name' oneself. Mark could do neither without stuttering.

My patient used fusion fantasies as a defence against knowing about the space between us. I experienced his speech as affectless monologues; I felt I was shut in, engulfed, enveloped. My patient in trying to describe how it had been with him and his mother described it as 'being in one skin'. My patient's stutter caused him most difficulty when he had to say his own name to introduce himself, that is to acknowledge his self, his own separate identity, that which his mother sought to deny as she sought to perpetuate fusion fantasies, for example in the promise she extracted each night about his dreams.

How did Mark's stutter arise? What did it signify in relation to his developing self? Sound-making communication begins as an entirely emotional experience located in the amygdala. In all children the right hemisphere is dominant for language at the beginning of life but by 5 years old dominance of the left 'thinking' hemisphere becomes securely established for the processing and production of language in most children. Brain scans offer evidence that for many stutterers the competition between the hemispheres is as yet unresolved (Ludlow 2000). Neuroscientists have also assembled research findings which make clear that right brain activity is a feature of those who have experienced trauma, and that those who have experienced early relational trauma, involving intrusion into bodily integrity are the most vulnerable. In Mark's case it may be that early relational trauma kept his attempts at sound making partially located in the right brain. (It is interesting to note that he, in common with many stutterers, had no difficulty in singing, a right brain activity.)

Schore (1994) stresses the importance of the child's affective relationship with his mother in the development of one-word speech, arising out of the affective interchanges with the mother being imprinted into the right hemisphere. Schore comments: 'The child's name is typically the first emotion word that the child learns . . . This particular word may be especially emphasised by the affect regulating care-givers in stress-comforting exchanges' (Schore 1994: 488). The right hemisphere remains responsible for the rhythm, melody and emotional colouring of speech throughout life. The mother's emotional unavailability may impair the gradually separating infants ability to develop 'inner talk'. Speculatively one might also wonder whether Mark's damaging early experience, encoded in his right brain, may have kept his attempts at sound making partially located there also.

The right hemisphere dominates the fear response to early trauma such as Mark must have experienced from the very beginning with his unpredictable and volatile mother. Moments when Mark sought in a healthy way to separate from his mother evoked stress in her. Such stress appears to have inhibited Mark and made him fearful of such separation. He did not see approval in his mother's eyes that would have enabled him to move confidently away from her. Although such conclusions must as yet remain tentative, it may be that the competition between the regressive pull of the early emotional attachment to mother of the right hemisphere dominant period and the later left hemisphere period of imprinting of the more independent toddler was not successfully resolved in Mark and became expressed in his stutter.

Stern and misattunement

Stern (1985) has suggested that it is by means of the mother's purposeful misattunement that the child gradually becomes aware of separateness. He noted that mothers intentionally over or under match the infant's intensity, tuning or behavioural shape and concluded that the purpose of these misattunements was usually to increase or decrease the baby's level of activity or affect (Stern 1985: 148). In manageable, bearable amounts, the mother carefully moderates such separating. Stern characterizes as 'non-purposeful or true misattunement' those times when the mother incorrectly identifies the infant's feeling state, or is unable to find in herself the same internal state (Stern 1985: 149). If the child's emotional needs give rise to a painful feeling state in the mother then she will miscue her child about that need, the child will develop a sense of danger about that need and will in turn miscue the mother (Marvin et al. 2002: 109).

The long-term effects of trauma

In episodes of traumatic interaction with a parent, or primary care-giver, the child's brain state will mirror or match that of the threatening parent. This has chilling implications when one thinks of the child's brain matching of the mother's dysregulated states. The psychobiology of trauma is discussed more fully in Chapters 5 and 6. Here we should note that the baby's first state will be one of hypo-arousal matching that of the mother. When the distress reaches an unbearable level and the hopelessness and helplessness of the baby's experience becomes intolerable then hyper-arousal will follow, leading ultimately to dissociation. Schore describes such dissociation as utilizing 'numbing, avoidance, compliance, and restricted affect, mediated by high levels of behaviour-inhibiting cortisol, pain-numbing endogenous opioids' (Schore 2003a: 67).

Identification with the aggressor is one possible outcome of such experience as 'spatiotemporal imprinting of terror, rage and dissociation is a primary mechanism for the intergenerational transmission of violence' (Schore 2003a: 287). Likewise the child who experiences the acutely anxious parent, or depressed, disconnected mother, will internalize those states of mind. These children may appear withdrawn, fearful, even frozen. In fact they are using dissociative defensive strategies to eliminate awareness of trauma in order to try to maintain some sort of attachment to the care-giver, an attachment that is inevitable when needs for nurture and protection are taken into account. The primacy of patterning in the brain-mind means that continued exposure to such states ensures that they become established at the level of the implicit as character traits. The same defences will therefore come into play in the consulting-room if, as children or adults, they undertake therapy.

Children who have been subjected to traumatic relationships learn in their very body to be wary and to defend against further trauma. In a study of traumatized patients Binet was able to demonstrate that 'the unconscious sensibility of an unconscious patient can be fifty times more acute than that of a normal person' (Binet et al. 1896, cited in Shin et al. 2005: 186). This hypersensitivity to stressors is thought to be the result of repeated experience of excessive and sustained cortisol secretion.

Kagan (2004: 35) cites Porges' (1996) description of the three levels of neurological response that may be utilized when a child becomes afraid; the optimal is the social nervous system, based on the ventral vagal system. This is the system that the child whose relationships with caring adults are 'good enough' will be able to utilize. However, children with poor early experience may only be able to resort to the alternatives underpinned by the sympathetic nervous system that is fight or flight. As Schore emphasizes, when neither of these prove possible the parasympathetic nervous system takes over, shutting down the overactivity produced by the sympathetic nervous system, leading the child into the shut-down, frozen state that mimics death. Kagan (2004) comments:

> Trauma-induced physiological changes are most damaging from conception and during the child's first years. The signs and symptoms of disorganized attachment and trauma become a way of life. And each recurrence of violence and loss confirms for the child that his or her world is chaotic and dangerous.
>
> (Kagan 2004: 39)

Terr (1994) emphasizes that some children, particularly if they experience one horrific incident rather than sustained trauma over time, never forget what they experienced. The abuse of others is sustained enough to cause amnesia. In reviewing the large-scale study carried out by Williams (1994) on memory in women with a documented and proven history of childhood sexual abuse, Terr (1994) notes again that those who were youngest at the time of abuse had the poorest access to memory but also that those where the abuser was a family member or known to the family were those most likely to 'forget'. In Williams' (1994) sample of over 100 women, 38 per cent had forgotten.

Jung emphasized the damaging nature of early trauma. He understood that it may lead to the defence of dissociation, by which he understood that 'the emotional significance of the experience remains hidden all along from the patient so that not reaching consciousness, the emotion never wears itself out, it is never used up' (Jung 1912: para. 224). Let us visit briefly the childhoods of two girls and we will see something of the way in which traumatic experiences may become embedded in the depths of a young person's personality, out of mind one might observe, yet struggling to be acknowledged one way or another.

Harriet

I would like to introduce you to Harriet, a middle-aged woman, who came plagued by severe anxiety and the constriction of personality that is the result of severe and very early trauma. Harriet came in to four times a week analysis because of increasing feelings of intense anxiety. Harriet heard herself often described by her mother as a difficult baby, the result of a difficult pregnancy followed by a difficult birth, a baby who cried too much, for whom she had not enough milk, who continued to be difficult to feed and who was labelled as 'a failure to thrive' child. Her mother's moods were volatile; she would hit out frequently without any warning, shouting, 'And if you're going to cry I'll give you something to cry for. Don't flinch away from me.' She remembers her relationship with her father as one of open hostility. Alongside the constant emotional abuse this patient experienced sustained sexual abuse from her father, with the involvement of her mother, from about 3 or earlier to 9 years of age, when this was detected by the family doctor and stopped. He arranged for her well-being to be monitored until she left home in her late teens when she found her parents' alcoholism increasingly difficult to tolerate.

In childhood Harriet had been solitary; she felt alienated from the world of other children, her depression and lack of confidence made the easy friendships of ordinary childhood inaccessible to her. Harriet described to me how as a child she sought refuge in books and films. Later she was to realize that, although she sought to escape into them, the ones that remained powerfully with her were the ones that reflected one or another aspect of her frightening internal world, formed out of experiences of abuse. Thus *Snow White* was terrifying because the Witch (mother) gave the girl poisoned fruit. *Alice in Wonderland* terrified her because Alice fell into a world she couldn't understand, where she almost drowned in a pool of her own tears. *Bambi* was horrifying as the forest fire (of her rage) killed the mother and left Bambi alone with the father. *The Wizard of Oz* was the most frightening of all because there the girl encountered a man without a heart. There were more gentle nurturing themes but significantly in these books someone other than the parents cared for the children. Harriet longed to be one of the children in *Ballet Shoes*, looked after by a kindly guardian and allowed to enjoy dance. *Children of the New Forest* again bore witness to a protector figure, and life lived in safety and peace deep in the forest while civil war raged outside. The saddest feelings were evoked by Ginger, the spirited horse in *Black Beauty*, whose liveliness and very being were almost destroyed by those who should have cared for her. It seems that engaging with these themes in this way enabled the child, whose abuse was so severe it was put entirely 'out of mind', to have a means of holding on to the unknowable while still permitting the dissociation that made living at home possible. As Harriet began to recover memory and to work with the effects of abusive experience as revealed through the transference she found herself no longer able to escape into the world of fiction in the way she had continued to do from childhood.

In her daydreams, Harriet lived in those other worlds that she encountered in her books. When occasionally she was taken to the pantomime, each time she found herself longing to be taken home by the principal boy and to be cared for as that being's child. I say 'that being' because in English pantomime the principal boy is an attractive likeable hero but always played by a woman. For Harriet the principal boy was a different being from both her mother and her father because 'it' was neither woman nor man. It also meant that as 'its' child she would not have to grow into either woman or man. In adulthood without being at all aware of it she actually retreated into what she later described with huge pain as 'neuter gender identity'. At times Harriet actually wished to become the principal boy. She could then become the hero and at the same time be neither masculine nor feminine. In the character of the principal boy she had found a way to imagine retreat into a role where she would have been able to cease to struggle with what it is to be human.

Sophie

Sophie was rejected at birth by her mother, who was convinced that her third girl child would be a boy. In the family she was cast in the role of the scapegoat, regarded as responsible for any trouble and punished for it. She became a solitary child who took refuge in drawing, which had to be a secretive activity because of her mother's disapproval. She also found an escape in her love of animals and the countryside. When the gardener attempted to abuse her at the age of 8 years old, she managed to escape but felt she could tell no one of the incident, for which unconsciously she blamed herself. She had a favourite lane where she went to daydream; there she would meet a character like ET. This character would comfort her by saying, 'Don't worry, we are like you as well, we also have to seem one way on the outside but are different inside'. This remark was made on a later retelling of the incident and reflected a growing sense of the validity of her internal self in contrast to the adaptive outer self that her mother had required. This girl, who perceived that she was totally unacceptable to her mother and not the son so much desired by her father, kept hope alive inside herself through her art. She broke down and came into treatment when her daughter reached the age at which she had her traumatic experience with the gardener. Her adult paintings arising from her childhood are referred to in Chapter 9 of this book and appear as Plates 4–9. These two highly individual accounts of rather different childhood trauma demonstrate the children's need to retreat from the dangerous world outside into the world of trauma-related pretend.

The damaging long-term effects of fear

Eigen (2001) writes movingly of fright in his discussion of Bion's understanding of the breakdown in ability to process feelings. I find his sensitive description entirely applicable to the effects of early traumatic experience and the way in which it undermines the child's theory of mind.

> The personality has undergone a terrible fright probably repeatedly, probably suddenly. It is likely that fright permeated the atmosphere the individual was born into or was a significant

dimension or thread or grain in upbringing. The individual was born into a frightened and frightening world, a world in which being frightened plays a significant role . . . Personality [is] congealed or collapsed around or into the fright . . . It spreads through body, the way it feels to be a person, through character . . . We are haunted by truths that are too frightening to think, endure and work with . . . once personality is set in the mould of terror, it is difficult to move on . . . *Selfdestructive superego* is steeped in and draws power from generalized, formless dread . . . Rage is fed by terror.

(Eigen 2001: 24–5)

I would suggest that the conservative, traditional, verbal, cognitive left-brain communication between patient and neutral, abstinent analyst is not on its own sufficient cure for the right-brain, affective, dissociated, intersubjective distress that is the outcome of early relational trauma. Rather, Davies and Frawley (1994) have the right of it when they describe it as consisting of 'unsymbolised traumatic experiences, with a primitive core of unspeakable terror, intrusive ideation, and somatic sensations that exist cordoned off within the patient's psyche, unavailable to self-reflective processes and the traditional talking-cure' (Davies and Frawley 1994: 21). They emphasize the patient's ability to 'painstakingly erect the semblance of a functioning, adaptive interpersonally related self around the screaming core of a wounded and abandoned child' (Davies and Frawley 1994: 21). They describe this child aspect of the patient as a 'fully developed, dissociated, rather primitively organised alternative self' (Davies and Frawley 1994: 67). They suggest the analyst must be aware of both the coping adult self and the hidden abused child in the patient who presents for therapy.

Significance for the consulting-room

Adults who appear in the consulting-room with difficult early experience as part of their history will manifest this in their transference to the therapist, revealing the nature of their early attachment. Although the degree and the intensity may vary, as trust is established with the therapist these difficulties will emerge and require understanding and adaptation of technique in order to allow the early experience to be worked with and the adaptive, coping and above all self-protective adult to feel safe enough to permit such a process.

It will become apparent as the reader progresses through this book that I regard the relational aspects of the analytic experience as one of the most important factors that can bring about change. Kagan (2004), in his exploration of how to rebuild attachments with traumatized children, draws our attention to the power of good parenting as 'promoting repeated positive experiences of neural connections over time' (Kagan 2004: 214). I would emphasize strongly that it is neither possible, nor desirable, to attempt to turn the therapy into a replacement experience for poor early experience, rather I am advocating a way of working that through the transference–countertransference relationship makes the exploration of past psychic pain possible in the context of a new and enabling relationship.

The 'holding' environment that the analyst seeks to create will influence the arrangement of the room: couch and analyst's chair need to permit the emotional space that is traditionally associated with analysis but should be placed in such a way so that if the patient turns her head, each may look at the other. This is because the gaze and gaze-away sequences characteristic of infancy, accompanied by the sound exchanges of 'proto-conversation', may be a significant part of the experience of the analytic dyad. This experience of looking, of gazing may be an important part of the therapy when one considers what neuroscience has revealed about the mirroring processes that go on between mother and baby. Gaze clearly plays a crucial part in the development of a sense of self and a sense of the other, and underpins all social relating that develops out of the earliest relationship. It has been suggested that some of the success of techniques such as Eye Movement Densensitization and Reprocessing (EMDR) is directly attributable to the opportunities for this engaged, warm looking at the other that neuroscience has revealed to be crucial in infancy.

It is symbolic holding, rather than actual holding, that preserves the analytic space intrinsic to the analytic process as well as facilitating experience of safe and containing boundaries. The issue of actual touch is a complex one and much analytic thought has centred round its abuse rather than its use in the consulting-room. Gerhardt (2004) suggests that for a baby 'being lovingly held is the greatest spur to development', noting that the mother's 'autonomic nervous system in effect communicates with her baby's nervous system soothing it through touch' (Gerhardt 2004: 40). Kagan (2004) reminds us of Crittenden and Ainsworth's findings that in childhood, 'withholding close bodily contact accounted for anxious and avoidant behaviour patterns' (Crittenden and Ainsworth 1989, cited in Kagan 2004: 17). This experience and these sorts of attachments may become manifest in the transference/countertransference experience of patient and analyst. For some patients the analytic process may be assisted if the analyst is sitting quite close to the patient, for others this may be overwhelming. If possible the analyst's chair should not be placed between the patient and the door; such patients may find it more difficult to remain in the session at moments of terror if they feel that the way of escape is blocked. The use of silence must also be managed carefully for as Cozolino points out, 'silence is an ambiguous stimulus that activates systems of implicit memory' (Cozolino 2002: 99).

Concerning analytic breaks, therapists should be aware that there is strong evidence that separation from those on whom we depend raises cortisol levels, and that early separation from the mother has been shown to increase cortisol levels, leading to the description of corticotrophin releasing factor (CRF) as 'the biochemical of fear' (Gerhardt 2004: 73). This particularly affects those with attachments that are less than secure. Gerhardt notes that 'recent crucial evidence has shown that children with secure attachments do not release high levels of cortisol under stress, whereas insecure children do' (Gerhardt 2004: 72). With patients where over-stressful early experience of separation, often because of early hospitalization of mother or baby, has become etched into the very patterning of the brain, and with whom a dependent transference has developed, analytic breaks will naturally be experienced as acutely painful, and as such require very careful management.

Some therapists have sought to explore, one might even say to exploit, Stern's (1985) notion of purposeful misattunement and to apply it to the later stages of clinical work where the patient's prime need is to experience safe separateness. However, any use of processes of purposeful misattunement with traumatized patients relies very heavily on the empathic capacity of the analyst. Too much too soon, or an inability in the analyst to find in herself the same internal state as that of her patient, may retraumatize the patient. Such retraumatization can result in immense pain that may cause kindling in a session (see 'Lucy' in Chapter 5) and an unbearable increase in shame that may cause the patient to withdraw from contact, from relationship and even from the analysis itself. In a sense none of this empathic, right brain way of working is new to those who, with Jung, have always valued the analyst's relation to the patient's whole being. What is brought to us by the research in affective neuroscience is the understanding of the changes in the brain that enable the patient to gain mastery over such early experience.

Conclusion

What is clear is that real traumatic events happen to children and the earlier these are the stronger their influence on the way in which children experience the world and the way that they relate to others in the future. In short they exert a strong influence on how children develop. Both children and adults who have experienced early relational trauma may or may not be aware of it, but such traumatic experience will have become the basis for 'conscious imagination, for dreams and for unconscious fantasy' (Knox 2001: 626). As such these experiences must unconsciously influence an individual's way of relating, and how that person's life will be lived. For me in the consulting-room the crucial question is perhaps not so much what actually happened to the child (though this matters and will affect treatment strategies), but how early the child experienced relational trauma, whether it was with the primary care-giver, what it did to the child, how the child was affected, what the child then made of it, and how that has affected the development of the child or adult who presents for treatment.

Chapter 4

Memory systems

The making of memory

Memories are made when a group of neurons fire together and make a particular neural pattern that remains after the stimulus has gone. Short-term memory may last a few seconds – iconic memory – or a few minutes – working memory – that is information held in mind for the needs of the moment, perhaps drawn from the experience of the moment, perhaps recalled from long-term memory for the task of the moment. Long-term memory may be explicit (declarative), that is it contains that which we are able to recall at will and recognize as memory from the past, or implicit, that is unconscious, storing that which is automatic, or emotional.

Explicit memory

Explicit memory consists of episodic, personal, biographical memory, the 'This is my life' of memory, and semantic factual memory, the 'What' of memory. Explicit memory content is processed by the hippocampus that tags time and place to memory, dealing with the 'Where' and 'When' of memory, ensuring its accessibility to consciousness in an identifiable form. Once the hippocampus has helped to establish the memory in the cortex (a process which may take about two years to complete), each individual element that goes to make up each memory is stored at the cortical site where it was originally received.

Implicit memory

Implicit memory includes the 'How' and the 'Emotion' of memory. Procedural memory stores the 'How to', the acquired skills that become automatic. This memory is processed in the putamen and cerebellum. 'Emotional' memory derives from emotional response to stimuli and is processed by the amygdala. Negative or traumatic feeling responses are particularly associated with the amygdala. Implicit memory comes on line earlier than explicit memory because of the earlier development of the right hemisphere, that is the hemisphere most closely associated with emotion. Segal (1991), describing Melanie Klein's work with children, commented that 'one gets a glimpse of an internal phantasy world like a vast continent under the sea, the islands being its conscious, external, observable manifestations' (Segal 1991: 19).

Implicit memory is the source of the deeply founded ways of being and behaving that govern an individual life. These hidden depths are the early established patterns, recorded in the implicit memory store of the early developing right hemisphere. These are then manifest in the patient's ways of being, feeling and behaving which become known in the consulting-room through the transference and countertransference. Davies summarizes the view of Janet (1889), one of Jung's mentors, concerning memory in the following words:

> Janet came to believe that the memory processes, the usual typical schemas for integrating new incoming information, provided the essential organising mental systems. When operating smoothly, most of these processes were out of awareness. These schemas are flexible, and there is a constant oscillation between the effect of new information in changing the internal structure of organising schemas and the individual's reliance on these schemas in order to create mental order and internal organisation.
>
> (Davies 1996: 557)

Jung's work with the Word Association Test had led him to suggest that pauses in the subject's reaction indicated the presence of an unconscious 'feeling-toned complex' (Jung 1934a: para. 201). There were many such pauses observed in the early analytic work. Jung described such complexes as autonomous 'splinter psyches', fragments, which become split off because of traumatic experience

(Jung 1934a: para. 203). Shin et al. sought to investigate the effect of complexes on implicit learning and found that 'complexes shown to disturb conscious cognitive processing in fact enhanced the attention of the subjects and their performance on an implicit learning task' (Shin et al. 2005: 175). Ekstrom (2005) concludes that this research emphasizes, as Jung did, the relative nature of what is conscious and unconscious, and suggests that 'when we include implicit learning in the equation, we are also permitting a dynamic conception of memory [and that we are] beginning to account for learning as the result of synaptic complexity' (Ekstrom 2005: 193) and the fact that 'the structure and function of the brain are shaped by experience' (Siegel 1999: 25, cited in Ekstrom 2005: 193).

Encoding and recall: scenes and themes

Much of our understanding of how memory comes to be stored arises out of the work of the cognitive neuroscientists who are interested in artificial intelligence. Ekstrom (2004) summarizes the work of Schank who offers an explanation of memory structures based on narrative. Schank suggests that 'we need to tell someone else a story that describes our experience because the process of creating the story also creates the memory structure that will contain the gist of the story for the rest of our lives' (Schank and Morson 1990: 115, cited in Ekstrom 2004: 668). These stories are encoded in neural patterns that the brain matches against new experience. Schank argues that the brain particularly notices new deviations from the expected (remembered) pattern and creates new refinements of the pattern based on the new experience that has been noted. Ekstrom (2004) draws our attention to further work by Schank and his team that identifies basic 'memory packets' which operate as storage forms, created without our consciousness awareness, 'one such packet organises scenes and since we remember in scenes, these . . . allow us to travel from scene to scene' (Schank 1999: 123, summarized by Ekstrom 2004: 669). It is suggested that another more complex group of memory packets deals with themes: these enable the processing and bringing together of scenes along with the integration of more abstract information. Schank draws attention not only to the knowing that is cognitive or emotional but also to that which is bodily and for the most part unconscious.

When recall is required the cortex reconstructs the memory and the memory becomes available for use. The experiencing of the remembering will add to the memory, the form of the memory will change, perhaps imperceptibly, perhaps in a major way because of the circumstance in which it was recalled, for example a particular aspect of an incident, or detail of an individual or place concerned in it may be the focus of the rememberer's attention at the moment of recall and again at the subsequent restoring of the memory. When its use is over for that occasion it is disassembled and stored in its individual elements again at the cortical sites ready to be reassembled by the cortex should it be required.

The work of both Rossi (2004) and Ribeiro (2004) stresses the value of dreams and the dreaming process in the consolidation of memory. Both emphasize the importance of the zif-268 gene, 'a learning-related gene capable of triggering the experience-dependent strengthening of synaptic connections' (Ribeiro 2004: 7). Ribeiro comments: 'Despite its short duration REM [rapid eye movement] sleep is capable of boosting memory consolidation by activating genes linked to synaptic plasticity' (Ribeiro 2004: 1). I suggest that the plasticity of the brain in response to the experiences of the day is a central aspect of this consolidation or reconsolidation, and that the analytic process as it revisits past experience, particularly where trauma memories are concerned, may take advantage of the reconsolidation process to integrate the modulated affect that is the result of the relational experience within the analytic dyad.

Illustration

The following narrative seeks to illustrate the encoding and retrieval of mildly disturbing memory and the distortions than can occur in processing.

The most spectacular storm I have ever experienced is occurring in the mountains around me as I write in a room overlooking Lake Bled. It will remain with me long after I return home. I shall associate it with writing this and visiting Lake Bled, thus allowing my hippocampus to tag time and place to this memory, placing it securely in explicit memory. The storm has lasted for at least an hour, thunder and lightning again and again causing the same neuronal connections to establish themselves as clearly defined pathways in my brain. The sense of unease that such a storm always causes in me is difficult to pin down. While my attention is focused on writing, suddenly a long forgotten conversation with my grandfather surfaces from when I was about 5 years old. It is the story of him taking a bath in just such a mountain storm, reaching out of the bath to shut the window and his wet arm being struck by lightning in the process. No wonder shutting the door to the balcony when the storm began felt scary!

The story had been forgotten long since, the emotion engendered by it had nevertheless lingered in amygdaloidal memory, reinforced no doubt when I experienced similar storms, and affecting the ways I felt and behaved in them. And now the storm is over and the lost incident is remembered and has entered explicit memory. As I mull it over I realize that the fragment of memory that has returned is of an image of my grandfather's arm at the open bathroom window in his home in England, not abroad where the incident actually occurred! And so I note that the memory as remembered is not an accurate in every detail 'snap shot' account but nevertheless carries the emotional truth of the experience with my grandfather. Did I remember because of the trigger of a storm abroad and a door that needed to be shut, as much as because of the writing? The sense of unease may reoccur but at least I will now deal with it as an adult with an adult's capacity to assess risk rather than the fright of a 5 year old told a story that was too much for her.

In order to write the above I have drawn on procedural memory (how to type), biographical memory (the where and when of my life), semantic memory (Lake Bled, lightning and its effects) as well as the amygdaloidal emotional memory that caused the sense of unease. My hippocampus will begin to process the recording of the experience of writing this passage (where, when) until it can get stored in long-term memory; at this moment of writing it resides briefly in my working memory. As I read about the storm again many months after I was writing at Bled, the experience represented itself in a series of scenes, which were followed by scenes of Bled in other conditions, as if my memory was sorting and differentiating as part of the process of recall. Gradually the associated feelings of that evening also returned, alongside my current thoughts about memory processing. I noted that I was no longer disturbed either by the memory of the storm or by my memory of the story told by my grandfather so long ago.

Traumatic memory

When early attachment experiences are traumatic, and especially when these traumatic experiences are repeated again and again over time, as can occur with the extremely insensitive, very intrusive or actually cruel care-giver, they become indelibly etched into the young child's very being. How does this occur, one might ask? Severe traumatic experience of any kind leads to heightened activity within the right amygdala that enhances implicit or procedural emotional memory yet inhibits the storage of explicit or declarative memory. High levels of endorphins are also produced in states of traumatic stress and interfere with explicit memory consolidation; high levels of cortisol circulate that have a further adverse effect on the functioning of the hippocampus, which tags time and place to memories.

Van der Kolk (1996) notes that the freeze response associated with states of panic interferes with memory in animals and suggests the dissociative response in humans may affect explicit memory in a similar way. Implicit or procedural memories are 'readily acquired without intention and retained forever without awareness, especially if they are linked to a coincident emotional event' (Scaer 2001a: 37). Knox (2001) argues: 'Implicit memory is the basis for the transference . . . the internalisation of actual people and real events in the world gradually produces an unconscious pattern of generalised expectations about relationships' (Knox 2001: 622). Experience of abuse, 'burned' into implicit memory, is known, yet inaccessible to thought; such deeply held ways of being and behaving set the scene for the transference, experienced in analytic work with these patients.

Traumatic experience affects both the encoding and recall of the memories associated with it. The earlier in life and the more sustained the traumatic experience is, the more likely this is to happen. Such traumatic experience becomes encoded in implicit memory, unavailable to the conscious mind. The body may hold the memory for the patient for many years until mind and psyche are strong enough to deal with the unbearable experience. Sometimes the trauma is manifest in symptoms which in a special way seem to point to the earlier traumatic experience.

Some degree of emotional stimulation makes encoding and retrieval easier, however if arousal is over-strong and stressful then explicit memory formation is likely to be impaired. Pally (2000) comments:

> Hyper-arousal of trauma functionally inactivates the left hemisphere of the brain, [eliminating hippocampal processing] leaving memory to be encoded primarily on the right [in amygdaloidal memory] . . . if the left side does not have the information, the person acts as if they don't know the information. Subsequently if an environmental stimulus triggers reactivation of the right-sided memory, the left processes it and the information is verbally recalled [thus making possible the recall of traumatic memory].
>
> (Pally 2000: 123)

Schore points out that even low-intensity interpersonal stressors beneath the level of consciousness can activate unmodulated terrifying and painful emotional experiences of an individual's early history that are imprinted into amygdalar-hypothalamic circuits. In these circumstances fear-freeze responses would be intense because they would not be regulated by the orbital frontal and medial frontal areas (Schore 2003a: 256).

The brain pattern matches in a rather general way in an effort to protect from further distress. This gives rise to the false associations and generalizations that analytic work seeks to explore; the transference/countertransference experience becomes the vehicle for modifying these. In the non-threatening situation of the consulting-room the transference can be experienced and analysed and the necessary stimulation to the cortex provided through the verbalizing involved in free association and response to interpretation.

Susan

Susan experienced a prolonged separation from her mother, a single parent, from the age of 6 weeks old to 18 months old, and then at 18 months old experienced the almost total loss of the single aunt who came and stayed in their home and who had acted as the primary caretaker during that time, until the family doctor became concerned at her serious failure to thrive and recommended that the aunt visit once weekly. At about 3 years old, she was again separated from her mother; this time she was sent to stay with cousins some distance away. She experienced abuse by her uncle, who she came to call 'daddy', while with this family. It is not clear how long her stay with this family was, and therefore how long she may have been subjected to abusive experience. She never told her much-loved aunt or her mother: her uncle had told her that if she told someone that person would die. She seems to have put the experience almost entirely out of mind.

This patient, a talented musician, discovered in analysis how as a child she had used music as a safe place to escape into, and how it became a shield, a means of defence against knowing about her painful early memories. She was particularly aware of the effect that sad-sounding songs had on her.

Panksepp (1998) notes that 'one of the most intriguing manifestations of separation distress in the human brain may reflect a powerful response many of us have to certain types of music'. He suggests:

> a major component of the poignant feelings that accompany sad music (what one might call the chill or tingle factor) may acoustically resemble separation distress vocalisations – the primal cry of being lost or in despair.
>
> (Panksepp 1998: 278)

A physical symptom in a patient may sometimes point to earlier trauma, while still helping to keep it out of mind. The body bears the burden (Scaer 2001a) and the body never lies (Miller 2005).

This seems to have been the case for Susan. Her love of music had been encouraged at her first school by the enjoyment of music that pervaded the atmosphere there. At 5 years old she loved the class singing lessons in which the teacher began to teach the children to sing, using tonic-solfa. On one occasion in order to help the children the much-loved teacher began to use a family of dolls. She explained that 'doh' was the mother in the family, next to her was 'ray' the little baby, next to 'ray' was 'me', a little girl doll dressed in green, the little girl's favourite colour. She understood 'me' to be 'me', that is herself.

Then suddenly the teacher was explaining that really the next note 'fah', the father in the family, was much closer to 'me' than the other notes, and that if you put them together it wasn't nice at all. I surmise that my patient's defences must have fractured at that moment and a kindling process began to occur in her brain. To the horror of the teacher the child went into her first grand mal seizure. When the child came to, her mother was there and she was taken home. She had no drug treatment and no further seizures until a stressful period in adulthood when she was referred to me. It was not until well into therapy that she was able to think fully about the abusive nature of her early experience and to link her shock at the teacher's description of the relation between 'me' and 'fah'.

Music was in some way a safe place into which she could retreat yet it also carried sinister echoes of the experience from which she sought to escape. In one session she explained that she loved early choral music because of 'its disembodied quality' but also spoke of the importance of the 'false relation' in the music of two such composers. She explained the way in which these notes that should jar because of their false relation to the rest of the music (much like her first teacher's description of the relation of 'me' and 'fah'), actually have a 'sizzling quality like wearing bright pink with orange'. We were able to use this description to begin to explore the difficult area of the 'sizzling' sexual feelings she may have experienced in relation to her uncle at the time of the abuse. Cozolino (2002) comments: 'What Freud called defences are ways in which neural networks have organised in the face of difficulties during development' (Cozolino 2002: 48).

I began to feel very guilty in Susan's sessions for, try as I would to remain attentive, every week I struggled with an overwhelming desire to sleep, such as I had never experienced before. 'Was it because her appointment was in the afternoon?' I asked myself. I began to wonder about the countertransference, because no other patient had affected me in quite this way. When she asked to come twice a week I made sure her second appointment was on a Monday morning when I would be at my freshest. But sure enough we would be ten minutes into the session and I would begin to feel the overwhelming sleepiness that I experienced with her in her afternoon sessions. The sleepiness represented my countertransference experience of her dissociative defence against allowing knowledge of her trauma. As the analysis progressed more of her feelings about this emerged in a series of dreams, a selection of which are presented in Chapter 8. She experienced repeated loss of the primary care-giver (first her mother, then her aunt, then her mother) at an early age and again in latency. She then experienced sexual abuse. She fought all her life to keep her loss, grief and anger, stored in implicit memory, out of mind. As the therapy progressed I became more able to look for the hidden signs of rage at the moments when sleepiness threatened, and my patient became much more able to express her anger with me, for example over times of impending separation caused by weekends and holiday breaks. When we were able to find a way to speak of her anger then immediately the session became more alive and my sleepiness vanished.

Modell points out that it is the non-communication of affects that induces precisely this sort of countertransference response in the analyst. It seems that it is often the dissociated affect that causes just this sort of countertransference response in the analyst. This way of dealing with dissociated affect not only may be defensive but also may re-enact the seeming indifference of earlier care-givers.

Many for whom trauma has been sustained over time lose memory of it. If the trauma is before 3 years old then the capacity to remember is not yet available. In the case of children of less than 36 months old the processing of memory is still very much limited to the right brain as the left brain development with its capacity for verbal processing and hippocampal processing of memory is not yet completely on line. Terr's (1994) 'True memories of childhood trauma: flaws, absences and returns' seeks to grapple with the problem that confronts all of us who struggle with the uncertainties that arise in both patient and therapist, not to mention the general public at large, as one struggles with that not remembered, half remembered, remembered only in patches, retained only in body memory yet portrayed in the transference and experienced by the therapist in the countertransference. Here I think that child therapists have the advantage: they are closer to the trauma and often the child has very clear ways of portraying it to the therapist.

Terr (1994) cites five studies of 'true' trauma experience in children and from these studies makes the following points. In those who had memory of their trauma, while the gist of the experience was remembered accurately, there were flaws of memory, both visual perception and perception of time were subject to distortion. In those where there was absence of memory in the face of true documented traumas it was clear that children who were under 28–36 months of age could not verbally remember their trauma but might have body memories or vague sense of foreboding when in a context which reminded of the trauma. Those older children who experienced abuse demonstrated that 'prolonged or recurring traumatic events would be less available to recall than a single short traumatic event' (Terr 1994: 74). Children who lacked trauma memory nevertheless demonstrated trauma symptoms (the most common of which were post-traumatic, repetitive play, personality change and trauma-related fears), 'the only factor linked to having no trauma symptoms turned out to be harbouring a false memory' (Terr 1994: 75). Terr comments on the absence of memory in those who experienced sustained and long-term trauma in terms of defence, suggesting that these children 'have mustered up their defences to hold their horrors in check' (Terr 1994: 75). She summarizes:

> Children old enough to remember their traumas may defend themselves from prolonged or repeated trauma by putting their traumas out of mind, deliberately 'suppressing' or unconsciously and undeliberately 'repressing' them. Traumatized children may also dissociate, teaching themselves to self-hypnotize and to enter planes of consciousness in which they fail to take in and register full memories of their traumas. Children may split creating good sides to themselves that know nothing about the awful experiences their cut off bad selves know. They may displace, concentrating deliberately on something similar but less cathected than the trauma, and, thus making their memories slip away. I have found that in my evaluations of adults who have lost parts or all of their memories of childhood traumas that all five of these defences can work against memory.
>
> (Terr 1994: 76)

Amanda

I would like to introduce Amanda briefly to you; I have written about the emergence of memory in her treatment more fully in the *Journal of Analytical Psychology* (Wilkinson 2003). Amanda remembers only a difficult relationship with her mother. She was one of three children. She felt that the other two children were special, in that her sister was pretty and was her mother's favourite girl, and her brother was special as the only boy. Her mother gave her a nickname which made her feel ugly and which was in strong contrast to the pet name given to her sister, which implied beauty. She loved her father and felt closest to him. One night when she was 6 years old, in bed in the room she shared with her sister, she heard her parents quarrelling violently downstairs as they often did. Her father came up the stairs, which she could partly see through the open door of the bedroom. As he came into her line of vision he fell forward, making a horrible noise, and collapsed on the landing. Amanda realized that she was sobbing and crept into bed with her elder sister. Her mother rushed upstairs, called out to the children to stop crying and slammed the girls' door shut. Amanda was certain her father was dead and indeed he had died immediately. Her mother admitted later that, in an attempt to keep the children away from the bedroom where his body lay, she had told them he was not dead. They were sent to school the next day as if nothing had happened. Amanda felt totally confused; she was sure he was dead. Later in the day she heard from children in the street that her father had died.

Her mother sent all three children away to boarding school soon after, telling them she had arranged this because she was going to kill herself. It was a school where every child had lost at least one parent, some two. Amanda was frightened about what her mother might do and desperately unhappy at school. She suffered constantly from eyes that were stuck together with infection: she would pull her lashes out as if she wanted to stop herself from seeing the plight she was in and to stop herself from beginning to cry. She was also plagued by itchy skin, something her father had complained of in the weeks before his death. She was unable to learn and left school with no qualifications. She married young, had children and later with the help of therapy was able to embark on higher education and a career.

The facts of her early distress related to witnessing her father's sudden death as a young child remained known to Amanda. She never forgot the noise her father had made. Her brother had found out that the sound frightened her and made it frequently to tease her and no doubt to act out his own feelings in relation to it. But she forgot much else from childhood and had no visual knowledge of what she had seen of her father's death. As she settled into therapy and began to have flashbacks and to work with them with her therapist, the therapist died suddenly and totally unexpectedly. Amanda said 'Goodbye' to her before a fortnight's break and then never saw her again. Some months later Amanda arrived in my consulting-room in a state of numbness, confusion and terror. It took many months for this to ease. On one occasion when I had a bout of coughing she became terrified I would die there and then. We worked with her feelings about my vulnerability for many months, especially over the breaks and the anniversaries of the loss and of the death of the therapist. Slowly but surely first the numbness and then the confusion eased, she became more able to think and was able to return to the dissertation for a higher degree that she had put to one side.

Patients who have been traumatized are hypervigilant and subject to flashbacks that may be triggered by a stimulus that in some way matches past bad experience and because the brain pattern matches to protect from a repetition of trauma, the patient becomes overwhelmed by an experience that has a 'here and now' rather than a 'there and then' quality to it. Eighteen months later Amanda felt able to tell me about a particularly frightening flashback that had occurred three years previously but which she had only just begun to be able to think about. She had been happily seated on a chair lift with her husband beside her, the two children ahead of them, going up a mountain. She remembered the loveliness of the day and the other happy families going up and down on the lift also with children, picnic baskets and pets on their knees. Suddenly she had become acutely aware of the angle of the slope of the mountain in relation to the chair lift and the scene took on a nightmare quality for her as she 'saw' picnic baskets, pets and even children slide off the knees of the travellers, followed by the travellers themselves. Her husband became aware that she was white and shaking; with difficulty she was helped from the chair lift at the top where she tried to explain something of what had happened to her anxious family. As she reflected on the incident with me Amanda wondered whether it could be that the chair lift passing over the angle of the slope had somehow replicated the angles she had seen of the stairs and of her father's falling body at the moment of his death. Until that moment, while she could remember the noise her father had made because of her brother's attempts to keep it in mind, she had not been able to remember what she had seen through the open door.

In the following weeks after recounting this and experiencing the feelings associated with it and with both deaths, my patient seemed much more able to engage with life. Two months later she reported that the feeling she had had, of being dead herself, had vanished with the telling of the incident and had not returned.

From an information-processing perspective, Brewin et al. (1996) present a dual representation theory of the effect of trauma on memory, one being explicit and verbally accessible, the other implicit and situationally accessible, automatically triggered by situational clues. Brewin and Andrews suggest that through repeated activation and entry into working memory flashbacks can become integrated with regular biographical memories (Brewin and Andrews 1998: 964–5).

The questions surrounding the recall of memory and accuracy of memories that surface in the consulting-room have been widely discussed. While the false memory debate continues, we should also be aware of the way in which the changing of emotional memory may actually be a benign aspect of analytic work, in that the retelling (from explicit) or re-experiencing (from implicit) of memories in the presence of the analyst may lead to a modulation in the quality of the affect associated with the memory, thus modifying the memory, in the case of the traumatic memory gradually helping to turn the unmanageable into the manageable.

Researchers are exploring techniques and drug therapies which may aid the forgetting of unwanted emotional memory (Miller 2004). Using fMRI scanning, researchers were able to show that when volunteers sought to suppress a memory the dorsolateral prefrontal cortex (seat of executive control) became active and activity in the hippocampus (a key memory centre) decreased. Trauma therapists may be setting a similar process to work when they encourage the PTSD patient with the persistently troubling flashback experience to 'throw the bad memory away' as it surfaces. A similar technique may be at work when children or adults recall a traumatic incident and are asked to tell it again, this time taking control, rethinking the ending, or in analytic terms telling the story and beginning to get some distance as they share it again in the safety of the analytic relationship. Scanning while these 'reappraisal' techniques were being used revealed that the prefrontal cortex lit up while the amygdala grew quieter. Miller (2004) notes that 'some studies have found heightened amygdala activity and decreased prefrontal cortex activity in depressed people ... that might mean depressed people are less able to tap into networks for reappraisal' (Miller 2004: 35). He notes that one small study revealed that ten sessions of transcranial magnetic stimulation (TMS) on the dorsolateral prefrontal cortex had a therapeutic effect on ten patients with PTSD. One might also argue that the talking cure to which 'reappraisal' is integral may also help to develop cortical control over amygdaloidal activity. Some advocate a drugs-based approach noting that memories of emotionally significant events are strengthened by stress hormones such as adrenaline. They argue that the use of drugs such as propranolol, offered to those who have experienced a sudden traumatic incident such as a rail or car crash, might limit the incidence of PTSD.

It has long been known that a certain amount of arousal with the resulting adrenaline rush that accompanies it will enhance memory. However, people are still puzzled and sometimes critical of those who, in extreme circumstances of hopelessness and helplessness that can accompany some traumatic or abusive experience, lose memory and remember only in the body until a particular circumstance triggers memory. Let us consider the quality of abusive experience and the likely effect on the patient's memory of it. The experience of being helpless in the face of danger brings into play all the most basic mechanisms we have in order to survive. This response includes the release of epinephrine and norepinephrine that enable the hypothalamus to activate the most basic defence mechanisms to ensure the survival of the individual and the species, that is flight or fight, and which heighten memory for the experience. As the sympathetic nervous system comes into play-energy-promoting arousal occurs, bringing increases in blood sugar, heart and breathing rate, as well as pupil dilation and increases in muscle tone and mental activity.

However, if the frantic distress associated with trauma takes its toll, and fight or flight is perceived to be impossible, hopelessness and helplessness supervene and the limbic system commands the freeze reaction. The parasympathetic nervous system takes over and inhibits activity, slows heart and breathing rates, lowers blood pressure, relaxes muscles and constricts pupils, in spite of the increases in adrenaline circulating as a result of the earlier phase of hyper-arousal. It is then that disengagement and dissociation of both mind and body occur. Such traumatic experience becomes encoded only in implicit memory, unavailable to the conscious mind.

LeDoux emphasizes the importance of the connections between the hippocampus and the amygdala in the contextual processing of fear (LeDoux 2002: 216) and suggests that 'if the degree of emotional arousal is moderate during memory formation, memory is strengthened. But if the arousal is strong, especially if it is highly stressful then memory is often impaired' (LeDoux 2002: 222). LeDoux also questions the dominance of the limbic system in the functioning of the emotional brain (LeDoux 2002: 210). He offers an account of PTSD which is based on direct projections from the subcortical sensory-processing regions that 'turn on the amygdala and start emotional reactions before the cortex has a chance to figure out what it is that is being reacted to' (LeDoux 1996: 257). He emphasizes the effect of trauma on the functioning of the hippocampus and suggests that in some instances at least this may be the cause of memory loss (LeDoux 2002).

Harriet

In contrast to Susan and Amanda, Harriet's early trauma seems to have been put almost entirely 'out of mind'. For Harriet a series of dreams led to a gradually dawning awareness of her traumatic early experience. I seek to demonstrate the way in which the total interactive, intersubjective experience in the analytic dyad as analyst and patient work with these dreams enables the development of the emotional scaffolding necessary for the process of trauma 'coming into mind'.

Harriet, a middle-aged woman, came in to four times a week analysis because of increasing feelings of intense anxiety. Harriet had heard herself often described by her mother as a difficult baby, the result of a difficult pregnancy, a baby who cried too much, for whom she had not enough milk, who continued to be difficult to feed. Her mother's moods were volatile; she would hit out frequently without any warning, shouting, 'And if you're going to cry I'll give you something to cry for. Don't flinch away from me'. She remembers her relationship with her father as one of open hostility. Nevertheless a loving aunt looked after her for one day each week and this relationship provided an experience of loving containment for Harriet. Alongside the constant emotional abuse from her mother this patient experienced sexual abuse from her father until the family doctor detected this and it was stopped. It seems the experience was then almost completely forgotten. The doctor arranged for her physical well-being to be monitored until she left home in her late teens, when she found her parents' alcoholism increasingly difficult to tolerate. As the analytic dyad became securely established, Harriet's experience that had been put entirely out of mind began to emerge in many vivid dreams that announced more and more clearly the theme of abuse. This powerful healing process felt to her as if it arose from deep within her; analysis of it made possible the retrieval of feeling and memory.

The first six months of the analysis was a time of increasingly regressive experiences in the consulting-room with both analyst and patient aware of a huge amount of 'unknown' early distress. Harriet brought many dreams that announced more and more clearly the theme of abuse. I include two at this point:

Dream 'You were too young'

Harriet was in a double bed in her bedroom that was decorated in blue, reminding her of her childhood bedroom. There was a roaring fire at the foot of the bed. The analyst sat in a chair at the foot of the bed. She said, 'Don't think this was for you'. Harriet asked, 'Why?' The analyst replied, 'Well, your age'.

Dream 'The wound can be healed'

Harriet dreamt of trouble with her right knee. In the past no doctor had been able to find the cause of the condition. Now she complained again and a new doctor at first thought it might be nothing, but on looking more closely was able to see something stuck in her knee. It turned out to be a T-square shaped razor that she must have knelt on at the time it first began to hurt. The wound had closed over and the problem had been hidden. Now the new doctor would heal it.

After about six months the analytic dyad decided together that an increase in the number of sessions a week would be appropriate. In the first session after they had arranged to meet more frequently, Harriet suddenly had a memory of herself at about 4 years old leaving the room, crossing the landing holding her father's hand and going into her bedroom. She saw her father's figure at the foot of the bed, blotting out the blue sky and then the metal buckle of his open jacket dangling in her face. In terror she moved up the couch to get away from the memory and back to the safety of the analyst.

Knox notes that at any time a patient may 'suddenly find him/herself vividly re-living the abuse in the most painful and terrifying way if something happens to trigger state-dependent retrieval' (Knox 2001: 620). Schore observes: 'In these flashback moments, a right subcortically-driven re-enactment, encoded in implicit memory would occur in the form of a strong physiological autonomic dysregulation and highly aversive motivational state of terror and helplessness' (Schore 2002: 29). He emphasizes how

> even subliminally processed low-intensity interpersonal stressors could activate unmodulated terrifying and painful emotional experiences of an individual's early history that are imprinted into amygdalar-hypothalamic circuits.
>
> (Schore 2001b: 227)

He concludes that dissociation reflects 'a severe dysfunction of the right brain's vertically organised systems that perform attachment, affect regulating, and stress modulating functions, which in turn impair the capacity to maintain a coherent, continuous and unified sense of self' (Schore 2002: 32).

A few days later Harriet dreamt a new version of a terror dream that had pursued her from childhood, but now its meaning was transparent:

Dream 'Pursued'

Harriet was in an upstairs room in a house she owned. Friends were in bed in other rooms. It was a frosty night so she put the

heat on. It melted the ice in the ceiling fittings. She ran effort-
lessly down the beautiful, curved staircase to a room where
children were watching adult TV illicitly. She turned the TV off
and went out into the garden. It was a dark night and as she
walked back to the house she realized it was raining. She could
see the rain against the lighted house ahead that now appeared
to be almost all glass, transparent. Suddenly there was lightning,
vibrating, straight lines of it. She feared she would be killed by
it. She crept closer to the retaining wall of the garden as she
walked up the drive. Again she feared the lightning might kill
her. She saw a man run out with a monstrous, huge oblong
piece of stone. He lifted it up. She thought, 'He'll kill me'. He
didn't see her. The man came closer. She thought, 'This is it,
now he really will kill me'. He raised the stone to hit her.
Nothingness.

In discussion it became clear that Harriet experienced the return of
memory as a series of jolts like the lightning flashes of her dream, felt
physically, and reminiscent of the partly remembered sexual act. The
unfreezing of thoughts frozen by a dissociative mechanism (that had
come into play to help her survive and which was remembered as
'escaping through the ceiling'), was pictured in the dream as the
unfreezing of the light fittings in the ceiling. Harriet felt that the
returning memory was retrieved in a way that was different from
ordinary memory and she described this process as 'memoring'.
Her memories tended to return in fragments each accompanied by
feelings of shame, horror and intense physical pain, either in her head
or in her 'tummy'. Despite the tears symbolized by the rain in the
dream, Harriet remained unable to cry. The pain of the countertransference was intense at this time.

Levin and Modell, cited in Pally (2000), have drawn attention to
the role of metaphor in facilitating the emergence of memory
because of its power to re-establish the integrated working together
of the two hemispheres of the brain after trauma. Pally comments:
'By containing within them sensory, imagistic, emotional and verbal
elements, metaphors are believed to activate multiple brain centres
simultaneously' (Pally 2000: 132). Harriet's dreams and Amanda's

vivid, visual metaphorical experience heralded the recovery of emotional memory of a dissociated event, the visual component of which was stored in the memory bank of the right hemisphere of the brain. The telling enabled something of the original experience to become available to the left. Affeld-Niemeyer suggests that it is 'not the recall of actual abuse that promotes therapeutic progress but the evolving symbolisations' (Affeld-Niemeyer 1995: 38). One would expect this to be the case if metaphor has such a radical capacity to promote change within the brain.

Conclusion

When implicit memory is realized in some way in the conscious mind, it cannot by its very nature return as a snapshot memory, or series of memories, of the actual event. It cannot return in that way because it has not been encoded in that way. The examples given in this chapter make clear how important it is for patients to process material held in implicit memory, but also how such memory, returning as it does in symbolic form, is inappropriate for forensic purposes. As Harriet commented thoughtfully: 'I agonized as early fragments of memory began to emerge. Fairly early on I found myself feeling that I must acknowledge what was emerging as the dynamics of my internal world whatever their truth or falsehood in reality'. Some of Harriet's memories that had been so frightening that they were dissociated emerged from the 'memoring' source in dream form. I must emphasize that it was her recall of the experience that had occurred when waking and remembering the dreaming, or talking about the dreams in the consulting-room, that became established in narrative memory and encoded in explicit memory, not the fine detail of the actual 'lost' experience. Chefetz reminds us that 'patients regularly report on previously not remembered episodes in their life which are profound in their implications' (Chefetz 1999: 376–7). With him, I suggest that 'we need to practice thoughtful uncertainty about what we hear, and model this for our patients, teaching them to tolerate not clearly knowing' while being able also to tolerate thinking the unthinkable.

Chapter 5

The fear system and psychological kindling in the brain-mind

> The explosion of affect is a complete invasion of the individual. It pounces on him like an enemy or a wild animal.
>
> (Jung 1928: para. 267)

In this chapter I will describe the fear circuit and will discuss affect-regulation in the analytic dyad in terms of quenching the kindling response in patients who have experienced early relational trauma and childhood abuse. In the clinical material that appears later in this chapter, I seek to demonstrate both the kindling response and the quenching of it in material taken from analytic sessions with two patients to show how analysis may actually change the mind, and enable development of the self.

Throughout this book I emphasize the importance of the quality of the early mother–child relationship in determining a child's ability to establish a secure base from which to explore the world in a confident manner. Eagle (2000: 126) offers a 'reminder that real traumatic events happen to children and that these real events exert a strong developmental influence on the way children experience the world and relate to others in the future'. He comments that it is this on which 'lives are made or broken' (Eagle 2000: 126). Traumatic experience inevitably determines the nature of the internal working models. Van der Kolk notes that trauma research has 'opened up entirely new insights in how extreme experiences throughout the life cycle can have profound effects on memory, affect regulation, biological stress modulation, and interpersonal relatedness' (van der Kolk 2000: 19). The experience of danger permitted by or even at the hands of the primary care-giver brings into play all the most basic mechanisms we have in order to survive.

The fear circuit

The amygdala's capacity to respond to danger produces almost instantaneous response in the body in the form of increased heart rate, respiration and blood pressure and enabling increased response from the musculature of the body. At the same time the cortex begins to assess the severity of the threat. If the danger is found to be negligible then the message to the amygdala quells the fear response. On the other hand, if the danger is felt to be so great that only 'playing dead' may offer a chance of survival then the parasympathetic nervous system will come into play and will damp down the overarousal initiated by the original fear response. Because this activity is essentially amygdaloidal in origin, it will be recorded in implicit memory and as such remain unavailable to the conscious mind, yet will be there to inform the fear response when similar threat is perceived at a later date (see Figure 5.1).

'Each of the glands produces and releases hormones into the bloodstream. The arrow shows the hypothalamic pituitary adrenal (HPA) axis, which controls the release of the stress hormone cortisol' (Gerhardt 2004: 60).

Both innate and learned danger signals can cause amygdala cells to fire rapidly, overcoming the GABA guard and initiating response in motor control areas. Because learning about danger is so important for survival the circuit is biased to react to stimuli associated with any earlier experience of danger, sometimes triggering a response that is not matched to the current environment, the reaction that affects patients with chronic PTSD. Once aroused in this way, these patients may remain so for long periods. The amygdala also receives modulatory inputs that reduce anxiety, for example serotonin fibres terminate there. Serotonin excites GABA cells and thus increases the capacity for inhibition of the panic response. Drugs like Prozac, which works by increasing serotonin levels, and Valium, which increases GABA activity, may reduce levels of anxiety (LeDoux 2002: 63).

Rosen and Schulkin (1998) hypothesize that

> during and following psychosocial stress the (normal) fear circuits may be over activated and a combination of behavioural and biological processes leads to the development of hyper excitable fear circuits ... turning the normal emotion of fear into pathological anxiety.
>
> (Rosen and Schulkin 1998: 325)

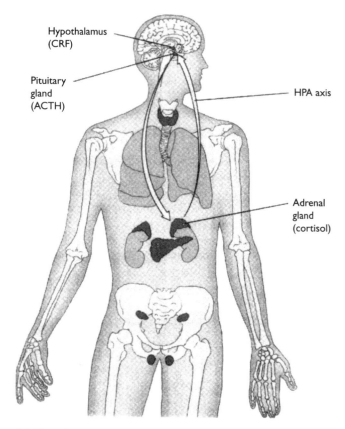

Hypothalamus
(CRF)

Pituitary
gland
(ACTH)

HPA axis

Adrenal
gland
(cortisol)

Figure 5.1 The release of the stress hormone cortisol

Source: Gerhardt 2004: 60

They note that

> the central nucleus of the amygdala may be important for cue-specific fear, the bed nucleus of the stria terminalis for non-specific fear, and the baso-lateral nucleus of the amygdala for both types of fear
>
> (Rosen and Schulkin 1998: 327)

They also emphasize that other brain regions, notably the hippocampus and the prefrontal cortex play a part in the processing and expression of fear. They conclude that 'theories that integrate the amygdala with many brain regions and systems are necessary for a full understanding of emotions' (Rosen and Schulkin 1998: 328). They emphasize that sensitization to stressors may become long lasting and difficult to treat, adding that 'indelible engrams are . . . formed in the brain' (Rosen and Schulkin 1998: 331). A study by Naccache et al. (2005: 7713) has indicated that even subliminal words can trigger long-lasting cerebral processes in terms of the amygdala's response to fearful or threatening stimuli.

Psychological kindling

Psychological kindling is the changed pattern of neuronal responses in the brain subsequent to emotional trauma whereby they fire in response to internal stimuli rather than external stimuli giving rise to flashbacks, epileptic seizures and nightmares. Scaer (2001b) notes the tendency to the freeze response that leads to the defence of dissociation in children who have been exposed to childhood sexual abuse and therefore their greater tendency to develop dissociative symptoms in subsequent experiences of trauma when adult. Following Levine (1997), he suggests that when the freezing response has been elicited in the face of irresolvable helplessness and remains unresolved 'persistent recurrent dissociation with associated endorphinergic reward might well potentiate the kindled trauma reflex' (Scaer 2001b: 76). Post and Weiss (1998) hypothesize that the recurrence of events which act as triggers brings about more severe and long-lasting consequences than isolated events, however disastrous. There may also be a kindling-like progression in the development of flashbacks, which may initially be triggered by cues linked to the original event and then begin to occur more spontaneously (Post and Weiss 1998).

Panksepp (1998) describes experimental research with rats that illustrates how powerful association may be. Following four baseline days of play, cat odour was introduced into the play chamber with the result that the animals continued to exhibit inhibition of play for up to five successive days. He concludes that 'cat smell can innately rouse a fear system in the rat brain, and this emotional system becomes rapidly associated with the contextual clues of the chamber' (Panksepp 1998: 19). While Panksepp urges caution in extrapolating to the human from animal research, he suggests that there are significant areas of overlap especially in the areas of basic motivations and emotions. Clearly cat smell is a species-specific fear but such research makes sense of the powerful responses that abused patients manifest in the consulting 'chamber' when contextual clues 'remind' of the abuse.

Research into the nature of traumatic memories was conducted using script driven symptom provocation, that is the production of a script which reminds of the trauma that is then played to patients while they are scanned. In patients with PTSD symptoms it revealed the development of a flashback type experience alongside significantly greater increase from baseline in heart-rate, as well as distinctly different connectivity patterns in the brain, to the response of traumatized patients who had not developed symptoms of PTSD. The PTSD patients showed a much more non-verbal pattern of memory than those traumatized patients who had not developed the over-reaction pattern associated with kindling and with PTSD (Lanius et al. 2004: 36). They urge further research into patterns of neuronal connectivity rather than specific brain areas will be essential to develop adequate understanding of the different anxiety disorders (Lanius et al. 2004: 43).

In the consulting-room, frequent states of hyper-arousal and the emergence of flashbacks may aggravate the kindling process (Post and Weiss 1998; Scaer 2001b). Affect-regulation therefore should become an integral aspect of the analytic endeavour. This means that the analyst will watch carefully for signs of psychological kindling and will seek to avoid the development of the kindled state in the patient with its inevitable release of a toxic 'soup' of chemicals into the brain. The kindled state, once aroused, may linger for some considerable time with detrimental effects to the patient's state of mind and general well-being. Cortisol levels may be raised resulting in damage to the hippocampus and the thalamus. How does the analyst help the patient to draw back from such a destructive inner process? Often it may help to begin to slow one's speech, to use a calm voice, often with a lower tone, speaking in what Williams (2004) has described as 'pastel rather than primary colours'. It may be that the therapist will make eye contact in what I can only describe as a 'holding' sort of way. The aim is not reassurance *per se*, or avoidance of the emerging material, but rather to enable the patient to remain 'in mind' and able to work. I specifically refer to symbolic 'holding'. Some colleagues working in related fields concerned with trauma therapy are exploring techniques that involve actual holding. In general, I do not believe actual touch is helpful in the analytic context because it may make it more difficult to preserve the symbolic space that is an intrinsic aspect of the analytic encounter. Colleagues who work in the field of trauma therapy emphasize that any use of touch, while having the advantage of accessing other pathways to the brain, requires very careful assessment of its appropriateness as patients who have experienced the physical trauma that comes from early hospitalization, physical or sexual abuse, or even in some cases unimaginative early handling, will be terrified by the concretizing of experience in the consulting-room and the very technique that was meant to assist may actually retraumatize.

One patient described her recurrent experience of being caught by a flashback as something that once begun, catapulted her into a parallel universe in an instant, much like Harry Potter's headlong rush towards platform nine and three-quarters (Rowling 1997). At such moments much will depend on the calm that the analyst is able to sustain in the face of much that urges consciously and unconsciously towards just the opposite. A lowering of tone and slowing of speech help to counteract the responses, triggered in the patient by the sudden flow of adrenalin, and experienced by the analyst in the countertransference. It may be possible to help the patient to modify their experience by use of a simple phrase such as 'it was then, not now'. Cozolino (2002) suggests that this is effective because it stimulates Broca's area and encourages the functioning of right and left hemispheres in a more integrated way. This process of cure is not initially that of making unconscious conscious, as with interpretation, rather it is the interactive experience within the analytic dyad that enables the development of regulatory capacity and reflective function. Fonagy argues that 'the ability to represent the idea of an affect is crucial in the achievement of control over overwhelming affect' (Fonagy 1991: 641). For this to occur successfully interpretations must be grounded in the emotional experiencing that occurs within the analytic dyad rather than being merely cognitive engaging primarily the left hemisphere alone. Beebe and Lachmann (2002) describe the analytic process as 'a co-constructed interactive process [in which] the narrative dynamic issues and the moment by moment negotiation of relatedness fluctuate between foreground and background' (Beebe and Lachmann 2002: 17).

'Kindling' in the analytic process: Lucy

The work in the consulting-room with its focus on the transference calls forth emotional responses that come from implicit, emotional, amygdaloidal memory traces that affect profoundly the individual's way of experiencing and relating to others. The more traumatic the early experience of the patient, the more necessary it is for the analyst to keep this firmly in mind. The analyst's way of working, of containing and moderating the affect evoked, will determine whether an experience 'kindles', that is activates an emergency response where no emergency is, releasing a toxic soup of chemicals in the brain and retraumatizing the patient or whether it facilitates the 'quenching' process which then permits analysis of the transference. LeDoux comments: 'Most of the time the brain holds the self together pretty well . . . if the self can be disassembled by experiences that alter connections, presumably it can also be reassembled by experiences that establish, change or renew connections' (LeDoux 2002: 307).

The difficulty of this work can be illustrated between an analyst and a patient who had experienced early and frequent hospitalization for painful treatment when she was less than 3 years old. Her consultant had been a man. Her condition necessitated further painful treatment at home. Such experience was for the most part inaccessible to her but was nevertheless retained in her amygdaloidal, emotional memory bank. Lucy was an only child whose father had died in a road traffic incident soon after her birth.

One very hot day as Lucy stood outside the analyst's house waiting for the door to be opened, the workman next door mused out loud to himself, 'Coca-cola? Oh, yes. That would be very nice'. Lucy surmised that he thought she lived there and was hoping that she would offer him one. She entered the consulting-room and told the story to the analyst with amusement.

ANALYST: Something we would all like.

The analyst thought it was Lucy who would like some coke, a good 'feed' in the session. She was picking up countertransferentially on something quite complex in that first moment. There was indeed Lucy's longing for a good session, a good feed before the break of the weekend. Somewhere at another level she sensed something different which evoked the opening remark she found herself making, somewhat to her own surprise. What she was not aware of was Lucy's intense dislike of coke, which she associated with hospital and her mother. Lucy thought it was the analyst who would like to be sitting outside drinking coke rather than working with her in the consulting-room. At an unconscious level, Lucy immediately experienced the builder as the doctor who made hurtful demands on her and the analyst as the needy and seemingly neglectful mother who drank coke in the hospital while Lucy experienced painful procedures. Although neither realized it at this point, the seeds for 'kindling' of traumatic memory to occur had been sown. Lucy switched from working on her own material to an attempt to care-take her 'needy' analyst.

LUCY: (*Lay down on the couch, feeling uneasy.*) I talked so much last time. I didn't leave much space for you.

ANALYST: Sounds as if that's said regretfully?

LUCY: No. Enquiringly.

ANALYST: We'll just leave it and see what happens today.

Lucy began to feel more unsettled and to look at the window and the garden. (Lucy, as a young child, had dissociated from the painful treatment she had experienced in her bedroom by an imaginary escape through the top left-hand corner of the window into the garden to play happily with the other children she heard out there.) Lucy looked up at the left-hand corner of the window, the look went unnoticed by the analyst but Lucy became momentarily aware of what she was doing. She did not tell her analyst, who unconsciously she was experiencing as an uncaring mother, who did not heed her distress. Instead she turned as she had done as a child to her own self-care system, without either being aware of it, what Kalsched (1996) described as the 'internal protector' had taken over. Unconsciously Lucy tried to halt the process of arousal that had begun.

LUCY: Is there a pond? (*She could see pond-plants. There had been no pond in the garden of her childhood.*)

ANALYST: Yes? (*The analyst was puzzled. She felt a sense of foreboding without quite knowing why.*)

Suddenly the workmen's voices were heard coming from the next house. The patient looked apprehensive.

ANALYST: Would you like me to shut the window?
LUCY: Yes, please.

The analyst got up and shut the window nearest to the workmen. The other remained open. Lucy began to move restlessly.

ANALYST: Would you like the other one closed?

Without waiting for an answer, the analyst found she had closed it. Surprised, she realized she was overcome by a sense of danger. She began to think but could not quite make the links that were necessary to understand what was happening. Both in the analytic dyad were experiencing Lucy's need to dissociate, to keep the feared happening 'out of mind'.

LUCY: (*Feeling increasingly uneasy*) Where's the picture with the woodland path got to?

The analyst felt very concerned. This patient had told her that she had run away down the woodland path, as a way of escaping from the room, in one of the most painful sessions they had experienced together. She gestured towards it, realizing difficult feelings were in the room such as those Lucy associated with the painting, and sought to imply this in her response.

ANALYST: It's still in the room.
LUCY: I need the blanket. (*She took it and covered herself. This alerted her to the difficulty that she was in.*) I need to understand what's happening.
ANALYST: Or possibly to allow it to deepen to see where it goes to?

Lucy felt terror and became speechless. The kindling process took over. The analyst became more concerned and tried to retrieve the situation, she began to speak of the past and the hospital room that the patient was in when she was little in an attempt to bring the patient's re-experiencing into something that could be thought about together. Lucy whimpered. The analyst continued to speak of Lucy's early experience, sensing her patient's speechless terror, she sought to find words for her. Lucy felt very small, about 3 years old. She sat up and looked across the seeming abyss at the analyst. At the same time she experienced a vivid visual fragment of memory of being in a drop-sided cot with black iron bars (a cot like the one she had slept in on repeated visits to hospital in the first three years of life). The drop-side was down but she could not get over it and out of the cot to reach her mother who stood some distance away, seemingly ignoring her struggles and remaining unmoved. She struggled for some way to put something of this into words.

LUCY: Could you move your chair a bit nearer?
ANALYST: No, I think we should see how we can manage.

On reflection the analyst might have chosen to move the chair a little while finding another way to confront the issues of power, control and helplessness that had been running through the material and which had culminated in this request. Alternatively she might have asked 'What would that mean?' or surmised out loud 'Perhaps you're feeling the need for holding and you are not feeling held here at the moment?' which might have opened up the transference experience to allow analysis. Perhaps if she had asked 'What's happening?' this might most effectively have enabled the patient to put into words the flashback that was overwhelming her. As it was, the actual comment was absorbed in a way that resulted in a full-blown experience that might well be described as psychological kindling. Lucy turned away from the analyst, withdrew into herself, holding herself rigid, knees drawn up in a foetal position, covered by the rug, thumb against her mouth, occasional tears trickling slowly from her eyes. (The patient had been punished for crying or sucking her thumb.) After some minutes she rubbed her forehead as if her head ached. Later she said she had felt as if she had experienced some terrible violation that she had been fighting to manage, fighting to dissociate, trying to get out of mind, to become mindless.

ANALYST: Are you trying to damp down your feelings on your own?

LUCY: I am trying to manage.

ANALYST: You insist on trying to survive on your own. Without me, although I am here.

LUCY: (*After a few minutes, speaks with some difficulty.*) That feels like a huge reproach. I am just trying to manage.

ANALYST: There are just a few minutes left.

Lucy sat up, folded the rug, moving like an automaton. The session drew to an end. In the next session Lucy reported that she had been very severely affected by the session both physically and mentally but had also become more clearly aware of the painful aspects of her relationship with her mother than ever before. Certainly for the analytic dyad it was an intensely painful transferential experience. While the tenor of the session was perhaps determined as the patient stood on the doorstep, on reflection the analyst regretted the 'kindling' that had caused such distress. A more responsive approach with the trauma articulated might not have led to the kindling experience that repeated old patterns in such a powerful way; whether it would have been possible to achieve this remains an imponderable.

'Quenching' in the analytic process: Harriet

Often the transference may turn the analyst into the abuser. In the process recording from part of a session that follows the kindling response evoked by the projection onto the analyst was 'quenched' by the right brain communications within the dyad. The analyst's face reflected and helped to modify emotion that threatened to over-whelm the patient. Harriet's early difficulties and the progress of the analysis reflected in Harriet's dreams are recorded in Chapter 4 pp. 71–4. Here I will just remind the reader that Harriet had a history of severe abuse within the family with little or no possibility of a healing environment, other than that provided by some contact with a loving aunt. The analytic process was fraught for the analytic dyad as kindling could occur. It seemed almost spontaneously at any moment, taking both by surprise.

Harriet begins to whimper quietly and looks increasingly fright-ened. She stares long and intently at her analyst. The analyst holds the patient's gaze. Her face expresses concern. Harriet continues whimpering, the patient continues to gaze into the analyst's eyes.

ANALYST: What is it you want to tell me?

Harriet shakes her head, looks confused. Holds her breath, then whimpers again. The analyst feels emotional pain, experiences physical pain in her lower right side and begins to feel sick. She continues to hold her patient's gaze. Harriet remains quiet for a while, then whimpers again. It seems she tries to speak to her analyst with her eyes.

ANALYST: (*in a containing tone of voice*) I know. (*Her face expresses holding.*)

Harriet's face becomes calmer. The whimpering ceases for a moment. Both faces become calmer. The corner of the analyst's mouth begins to express the hint of a smile. Harriet looks at her analyst's mouth and eyes. Begins to smile back. The whimpering stops. Her eyes clear. After a silence she says, 'What was that about?' The analyst replies, 'We don't know yet'.

That night the patient dreamt the fuller version of her recurrent childhood nightmare with detail that indicated the likelihood of abuse (presented in Chapter 4). Next day she brought the dream to analysis and was able to begin to discuss it in relation to her whimpering little child self. I consider the exchange recorded here to be illustrative of the work that takes place before the necessary analytic process of verbalization that followed in the subsequent session. Perhaps the former might be considered to be a form of 'proto-symbolization'.

In several sessions Harriet was to say in fright: 'Don't let Daddy come in here. Please don't let Daddy come in here'.

There are several responses one might make to this plea. My concern here would be to help to undo the dissociation, without provoking the kindling response. This becomes possible because the feelings are experienced and contained by the analyst.

HARRIET: (*Beginning to sound frightened*) Please don't let Daddy come into the room.

ANALYST: We'll do what has to be done.

This might be experienced as quite persecutory, and I am in danger of being perceived as all-powerful and abusive. My tone of voice may be perfectly acceptable to many patients but for these patients who are both fragile and hypervigilant it may be too strong. The tone used will be crucial in that it needs to 'hold' the patient and yet acknowledge how very frightening the original situation was, and the undoing of it is.

Or, ANALYST: You're quite safe here. (*This reassurance avoids the issue.*)

Or, ANALYST: It sounds as if it was very frightening if Daddy came into the room.

This begins to undo the dissociation; it helps the patient to begin to allow the dissociated contents into mind. Countertransferentially, I may find it difficult to make such a comment because of the patient's dissociative defence against pain.

Later I may wish to comment: 'That was then, not now'. (This might be appropriate towards the end of the session when some of the dissociation has been undone, and the 'then' and 'now' need to be differentiated in order to enable the patient to leave with a feeling of being contained.)

This work clearly poses some major difficulties. The earlier example of the work with Lucy may be understood in Stern's (1985) term as true misattunement where the analyst was not able to find in herself the same internal state as that of her patient and simply thinking about her patient was not enough because she did not have sufficient information, from her patient or from her countertransference, to understand what was happening in the room. How then do we avoid such hazards while managing the question of abstinence and distinguishing between libidinal wishes and developmental needs? How do we deal with our own desire to nurture, which these patients call forth so powerfully, without getting caught up in unhelpful countertransferential acting-out? How do we deal with the question of our own needs, for example with regard to breaks? How do we help the patient to manage the sudden descents into overwhelming distress and intensity of emotion associated with abuse, the seeming inability to escape from it, and the concomitant experience of the analyst as the abuser, and the unhelpful endorphinergic reward that may become enacted in the consulting-room? Where there is an early history of such traumatic experience, Schore suggests, 'small disruptions associated with interpersonal stresses too easily become rapidly amplified into intense distress states' (Schore 2001c: 228).

> The remarkable capacity of the brain to take a specific event and generalize, particularly with regard to threatening stimuli, makes humans vulnerable to the development of false associations, and false generalizations from a specific traumatic event to other non-threatening situations.
>
> (Perry 1999: 17)

Ferro suggests that microfractures in communication between analyst and patient are vital because they allow the transference to become 'the engine of the analysis, by contributing raw material from the patient's internal world and history'. He argues that it is essential that the analyst's mind has a 'semi-permeable quality, so that it can receive without being – excessively – invaded' (Ferro 2005: 34).

Howes suggests that as the experience that the patient is reliving emanates from what has been termed the emotional brain so the analyst must remain 'right brain, limbic' to achieve this empathy, while also remaining able to think (N. Howes, unpublished communication, 2000). Schore (2001b) comments:

> In the light of the central role of the limbic system in both attachments and in 'the organization of new learning', the corrective emotional experience of psychotherapy, which can alter attachment patterns, must involve unconscious right brain limbic learning.
>
> (Schore 2001a: 317)

The analyst who seeks to work in this right brain, limbic way is creating a dyadic experience that mirrors early infant–mother inter-action. Chu (1998) warns that 'passivity and withholding on the part of the therapist allow traumatic transferences to flourish'

(Chu 1998: 122). Lengthy silences also feed the traumatic transference for patients who have experienced early relational abuse. Chu warns that 'such transferences have their origins in a past reality and can rapidly become functionally psychotic' (Chu 1998: 122), much as we saw in the material from Lucy. Rather a willingness to engage the patient and to respond to the patient's gaze may be an integral part of such an analytic encounter, as demonstrated in the material from Harriet. Chu (1998) elucidates:

> Traditional psychoanalytic distance is designed to encourage transference distortions that are useful in breaking through the armour of well-defended persons in order to examine underlying feelings and attitudes. In contrast many abuse survivors have only brittle defences that shield against overwhelming and disorganizing underlying affects. Thus . . . therapy should generally attempt to *minimize* transference distortions.
>
> (Chu 1998: 122, italics author's own)

The arrangement of chair and couch, or chair and chair, must permit both gaze and 'gaze-away' behaviours that are part of normal mother–infant interaction. Schore (2001b) warns that rapid and intense right brain to right brain affective communications occur at levels beneath conscious awareness. He stresses the value of attention to the micro moment noting that tracking of 'very rapid affective phenomena in real time involves attention to a different time-scale than usual' (Schore 2001b: 71). He suggests that the analyst may learn most from 'the emotional tone of voice, small movements of facial muscles, spontaneous gestures and gaze aversions [of the patient]' (Schore 2001b: 70). Brown (2001) notes that 'it requires a finely attuned consciousness to discern and comprehend such changes within the body which are also the signal to changes in the psyche' (Brown 2001: 137). As a patient experiences the extreme distress engendered by a vivid revisiting of trauma, such moments of intense gaze may be used by the patient first to convey the intensity of her distress, and then by the analyst through subtle change of facial expression to modify and regulate the affect, before either become able to access the left brain and to begin to put words to such pain-filled experience. Brown describes just such pain-filled work in her account of therapy with a 10-year-old girl. She found that she learned

> To attend to my own body as an instrument of awareness and

knowing; to endeavour to become finely attuned to my own physical sensations and reactions as resonances of psychic contents not yet available to conscious thought; to value and to use my body as a means of registering and recognising the countertransference.

(Brown 2001: 145)

Analytic 'holding' through such moments is perhaps the most potent vehicle for healing, but such symbolic holding is sometimes one of the most important aspects of the therapy for such a patient needs to know that the early boundary violations that gave rise to so much trauma will not recur in analysis, while at the same time being impelled from within to test this to the limit. Therapists may be tempted to be drawn in to a re-enactment of the earlier abusive experience, especially if they become over-identified with the patient, or caught up in a wish to reparent the patient. Sidoli (2000) warns that

> when the analyst relinquishes the analytic attitude and is drawn into action by responding to the patient's body demands (by acting out sexually or in any other way), the analyst is repeating the early mother's behavior, that is to say not attending to the patient's emotional need and pain. Thus, the patient's potential for symbolic development is lost again and may be permanently impaired.
>
> (Sidoli 2000: 116)

McCann and Colletti (1994) have described the relationship of the analyst and the patient who has experienced early childhood abuse as a 'dance of empathy', choreographed and 'guided by the quality and consistency of the empathic responses, as determined by the therapist's counter transference' (McCann and Colletti 1994: 119). In the analytic 'dance' the patient may experience his or herself as the victim, perhaps as the result of too penetrative a transference interpretation that is then experienced as an attack. The patient will then experience the analyst as the persecutor, the analyst may sense this and attempt to step back. The patient then experiences this as a loss of empathy and the analyst becomes more like the mother who fails to protect. When the patient is in a dissociated state, often as a defence against the imagined abuser, then the analyst may feel like the victim child left alone in the room. Experiencing the analyst like this may provoke the abuser in the patient. Realization of this brings horror and shame and anger. Often the anger can be experienced only in projection and once again the analyst is experienced as the abuser, indeed the unwary may become just that under such intense transferential provocation. At times the sense of the patient's shame and humiliation might mean that the analyst wishes to rescue the patient, and so the dance moves on.

Brown (2001), describing her work with an adult patient, abused as a child and currently in an abusive relationship, emphasizes her own awareness of 'the abuse as a terrifying force, with the power to wreak appalling destruction; the exhausting struggle to maintain a defensive position in the face of that kind of energy' (Brown 2001: 149). Both analyst and patient will experience the force of the abuse and the defensive struggle as the transference/ countertransference experience oscillates between abuser and abused. McCann and Colletti (1994) warn that 'numbing, dissociation, fascination, revulsion, rescuing and blaming experienced in the countertransference can cause empathic strain and accompanying feelings of helplessness, rage, rescue and sadism [in the analyst]' (McCann and Colletti 1994: 90). Trowell (1998) describes her countertransference with one young patient: 'my reactions were very powerful and at times difficult to cope with: despair, fear, guilt, anger, the seduction of being the good, idealised, abandoning mother – the ease with which I could have been the cruel, sadistic foster-mother' (Trowell 1998: 162). Everest (1999) warns of the need for the analyst to be aware of his or her 'own mechanisms of dissociation' (Everest 1999: 459) in order to work successfully with dissociated patients. Clark (2001) warns: 'The persecuting soma often gets defensively projected or injected into the analyst [who] feels physically attacked from within as well as from without' (Clark 2001: 107). Davies and Frawley (1994) describe the analyst's countertransference responses as 'the map guiding the clinician through the hidden shoals of the transference' (Davies and Frawley 1994: 152). Perhaps if the countertransference is the map, the supervisor, internal, external or both, may be likened to the pilot, whose aid may well prove essential.

Sullivan and Gratton observe that 'electrophysiological and metabolic evidence supports the notion of excessive activation of right frontal systems in anxious states' (Sullivan and Gratton 2002: 107). They conclude that 'the notion of *normalising imbalances* of pre-frontal function in stress-related psychopathology must be considered central to successful therapies' (Sullivan and Gratton 2002: 107, italics in original).

Conclusion

Understanding the process of kindling and quenching in the way I have outlined enables the therapist to engage appropriately with the patient's affect and to modulate the extremes of over-arousal that may occur. Paying attention to affect in this way encourages a state of mind in the patient that makes possible the work of coming into mind. This approach enables the left-brain analytic processing, vital to a rebalancing process, that 'allows for the structural expansion of the patient's orbito-frontal system and its cortical and subcortical connections' (Schore 2001b: 72) and that strengthens cortical control over the amygdala (LeDoux 1996: 268).

Chapter 6

Un-doing dissociation

As a result of some psychic upheaval whole tracts of our being can plunge back into the unconscious and vanish from the surface for years and decades ... disturbances caused by affects are known technically as phenomena of dissociation and are indicative of a psychic split.

(Jung 1934b: para. 286)

The real emotional significance of that experience remains hidden all along from the patient, so that not reaching consciousness, the emotion never wears itself out, it is never used up.

(Jung 1912: para. 224)

Trauma needs to be undone in the brain. Although the self is fundamentally associative and relational, dissociative defences may come into play to protect a patient from overwhelming affect at a time when it would be truly unbearable. Their effects lie symbolically between 'in mind' and 'out of mind'. They hint at the truth, ready for the moment when the patient has sufficient ego strength to begin to confront it. Fonagy argues that 'the ability to re-present the idea of an affect is crucial in the achievement of control over overwhelming affect' (Fonagy 1991: 641). Achievement of this must be a major part of the analytic process with certain patients.

Working in Paris towards the end of the nineteenth century, Janet was the first to propose that traumatic memories may become split off, stressing that extreme emotional arousal might result in effects of trauma lingering on in an unintegrated way because they had never been able to be processed adequately. Freud and Jung studied in Paris, embraced dissociationist theory and wrote convincingly in support of it. Jung commented:

> As a result of some psychic upheaval whole tracts of our being can plunge back into the unconscious and vanish from the surface for years and decades ... disturbances caused by affects are known technically as phenomena of dissociation, and are indicative of a psychic split.
>
> (Jung 1934b: para. 286)

Jung warned that the real emotional significance of a childhood traumatic 'experience remains hidden all along from the patient, so that not reaching consciousness, the emotion never wears itself out, it is never used up' (Jung 1912: para. 222). He elucidated: 'A traumatic complex brings about the dissociation of the psyche. The complex is not under the control of the will and for this reason it possesses the quality of psychic autonomy' (Jung 1928: para. 266). He described such complexes as 'autonomous splinter psyches', fragments, which became split off because of traumatic experience (Jung 1934a: para. 203). Jung warned how the traumatic complex may suddenly return to consciousness, commenting, 'it forces itself tyrannically upon the conscious mind. The explosion of affect is a complete invasion of the individual. It pounces upon him like an enemy or a wild animal' (Jung 1928: para. 267). Later, as Freud and Jung began to place greater emphasis on fantasy and the inner world respectively, the effects of adverse external experience were belittled. Rather psychoanalysts and analysts sought to understand the roots of internal object relations within the psyche. However, the work of trauma theorists and therapists has led to renewed emphasis on Jung's earlier perspective that real, overwhelmingly traumatic, events might disappear from the mind and be held only in the unconscious, in implicit memory, in the forms of complexes.

The *Diagnostic and Statistical Manual of Mental Disorders* (DSM-IV) identifies dissociation as 'a disruption in the usually integrated functions of consciousness, memory, identity or perception of the environment' (American Psychiatric Association 1994). Schore (2005) argues the need for a fuller definition of dissociation that takes in awareness of the bodily and emotional aspects of dissociation that are so well documented today. He notes that the International Classification of Diseases (ICD-10) makes reference to 'a partial or complete loss of the normal integration between memories of the past, awareness of identity and immediate sensations and control of body movements' (World Health Organization 1992, cited in Schore 2005, in press) and that Spiegel and Cardena's (1991) widely used definition of dissociation as a 'structured separation of mental processes (e.g. thoughts, emotions, conation, memory and identity) that are ordinarily integrated' also includes the emotions (Spiegel and Cardena 1991: 367, cited in Schore, in press). Chefetz describes the fluctuating states of self-awareness that occur in the experience of the dissociative patient as alternating subjectivities that may exist without dissonance because of the particular nature of the dissociative defence (Chefetz 2000: 290). The multiplicity of definitions of dissociation reflects the complexity of what analysts may experience as they seek to work with patients who dissociate.

Chefetz notes that reports of persons with dissociative adaptations tend to have more non-verbal content (Chefetz 2000: 289). I understand this non-verbal content to be content originating predominantly from the activity of the right brain and from implicit memory, and indeed research has highlighted the differences in brain connectivity between those who have experienced trauma and have gone on to develop PTSD with those who have experienced trauma without developing the symptoms of PTSD. Lanius et al.'s use of fMRI scanning reveals greater activity in the right posterior cingulate gyrus, right caudate, right parietal lobe and right occipital lobe. They suggest that it is the patterns of connectivity in the brain that lead to the predominance of non-verbal recall in those with PTSD (Lanius et al. 2004: 36).

Chefetz asserts that awareness of the differing states of subjectivity experienced by these patients will allow work to take place through which affect can be contained and explored (Chefetz 2000: 289). This emphasis on alternating or differing states of subjectivity allows for the whole spectrum of experience of self and other. It embraces the differing states of subjectivity that we all experience as we function in relation to loved ones, to colleagues or to friends or indeed the way we will relate to any of these in differing ways depending on our external or internal transient experience. The spectrum continues on a scale that moves through the varied experiences presented by dissociative patients right through to the most pathological states encountered in work with patients in severe dissociative states.

The dissociative response to trauma may be expressed as it was experienced, in the entire psyche-soma entity. The work of a growing number of researchers attests to the detrimental long-term effects of exposure to traumatic stress, particularly stress in early childhood, stress that is sustained over a long period, and recurrent experience of traumatic stress (Schore 1994, 1996, 2001a, 2001b, 2003a, 2003b; van der Kolk 1996; Yehuda 1998; Teicher 2000, 2002; Scaer 2001a, 2001b). Stress hormones affect not only the brain but also the whole body, thus brain changes engender body changes. Grillon and colleagues note that the neurobiological response to stress produces long-lasting alterations in multiple neurochemical systems and that these adaptive alterations are 'idiosyncratic . . . and are influenced by innate characteristics as well as past experiences' (Grillon et al. 1996: 279). Chu notes that stress-responsive neurohormonal systems have been implicated in the development of PTSD: catecholamines (adrenaline, noradrenaline and dopamine, that enable and modulate bodily arousal in response to stress) and hormones involved in the hypothalamic pituitary adrenal axis (corticotrophin releasing factor, adrenal corticotrophic hormone (ACTH) and glucocorticoids) (Chu 1998: 55). The effects of continual exposure to such stressors may lead not only to PTSD but also to other bodily changes. For example, cortisol levels will be elevated initially with possible adverse effects, including cell death, in areas such as the hippocampus that are high in glucocoticoid receptors. However, the long-term effects of trauma are thought to result in lowered cortisol levels, which in turn may affect the body's immune system (Yehuda 1998: 97). Solomon understands the body as the location of early traumatic memories, arguing that because traumatic experience often happens early in life in many cases,

> The psyche is . . . unable to process it and is liable to store trauma in body memory . . . The patient's body has had to share the burden of the traumatising experience with the psyche. It is as if the psyche could not tolerate the full impact, or else could not make sense of the experience except by rendering it into organic form, or because the traumatising history had such real toxic effects on the physical system.
>
> (Solomon 2004: 649)

Scaer (2001a) lists a multiplicity of bodily symptoms, of unknown cause, that may be suffered by those who have experienced traumatic stress. He mentions neuromuscular symptoms, fibromyalgia, chronic fatigue syndrome, headaches, migraines, asthma, gastro-intestinal complaints, inflammatory bowel symptoms, pelvic, low back and bladder pain. He comments that 'when one is locked into ... adherence to Cartesian dualism, such syndromes defy explan-ation' (Scaer 2001a: 134). However, when understood as memory contained only in the body as a result of dissociation then treatment can be tailored to address the dissociative split, not just the bodily condition.

Dealing with the level of anxiety engendered by trauma of all kinds consumes considerable energy with significant psychological and biological consequences to the individual concerned (Rosen and Schulkin 1998). However, increased levels of energy and cre-ativity may be dramatic in patients whose treatments successfully address trauma-related anxiety. Scaer suggests that because the internal events in trauma become self-driven and self-perpetuating so the diseases associated with trauma

> reflect regulatory impairment, both sympathetic and para-sympathetic, with a predominance of vagal and parasympa-thetic syndromes in the later stages. [He notes that] conditioned imprinting of pain in procedural memory ... implies that trauma will have occurred in a state of helplessness without opportunity for spontaneous resolution of the freeze response.
> (Scaer 2001b: 85–6)

Early brain development is adversely affected by dissociative experience in the earliest relationships. Perry et al. emphasize that 'because the brain organises and internalises new information in a use-dependent fashion ... acute adaptive states, when they per-sist, can become maladaptive traits' (Perry et al. 1995: 271). Bromberg (2003) describes the experience of psychic trauma as that which floods the mind in an overwhelming way and is therefore unintegratable. He warns:

> this unintegratable affect ... threatens to disorganise the internal template on which one's experience of self-coherence, self-cohesiveness, and self-continuity depends ... The unprocessed 'not-me' experience held by a dissociated self-state as an affective memory without an autobiographical memory of its origin 'haunts' the self.
> (Bromberg 2003: 689)

Kalsched (1996) has described a similar process; he suggests that part of the patient grows up too soon and develops into a coping false self, much as Winnicott suggested, and part of the patient remains too young; experienced as 'the child', the true self remains hidden deep within the personality. He argues that recall of actual abuse stimulates archetypal images and notes that a powerful protector/persecutor figure (much like a harsh super-ego) is often encountered within the structure of the personality who actively seeks to guard the self from annihilation, even long after the danger is past. I understand these images as attempts of the mind to represent those experiences that have remained encapsulated in implicit memory (Kalsched 1996). Rosenbaum (2002), cited in Bromberg (2003: 707), finds a different image to describe the defence of the dissociative sufferer of trauma.

> Shutting the door of your own home won't make it safe. But maybe you can shut the door on yourself. Hide in one of those rooms, maybe even in the attic. Crawl inside and take cover from the hurt. After a while, with any luck, no one will even notice that you have been gone . . . All that's left to decide is when, if ever, to reemerge.
>
> (Rosenbaum 2002: 149)

Affeld-Niemeyer (1995: 37) observed of such patients: 'It is as if the soul stopped breathing'. To me it seems as if for many of the patients affected by early and sustained relational trauma that deep inside there is a frozen wasteland, a disintegrative state of frozen self, inhabited by both terrorist and terrorized, abuser and abused. This inner being is in a state of deep freeze, waiting for emotional supportive circumstances that will enable the thaw. This inner being is masked by an adaptive outer self where deintegrative and reintegrative processes still hold sway, through which the coping self developed, that enables the patient to manage. As therapy progresses, so slowly and painfully the thaw begins.

Traumatic experience affects both the encoding and recall of the memories associated with it. Perry (1999) observes that 'a pattern of incoming sensory information may be interpreted as danger and acted upon in the brain stem, midbrain and thalamus milliseconds before it gets to the cortex to be interpreted as harmless' (Perry 1999: 18). Peter Levine (1997) has described how in extreme situations feeling, sensation, behaviour, image and meaning become dissociated from one another. When the different elements of an unbearable experience get dissociated or split off from one another there can be no proper memory of the event. It will not be processed by the hippocampus, which tags time and place to memories, and so it cannot be stored as explicit or narrative memory. It cannot be recalled in the ordinary way because it has not been remembered in the ordinary way. Instead it will be encoded implicitly in the emotional brain and in the body to remind and warn when similar danger should threaten again.

Mollon reminds us that 'linkage may be severed between one area of awareness and another, between memory and affect, and between experience and identity' (Mollon 2002: 187). Sidoli suggests that such patients use their body as 'a container and signifier, as a kind of stage upon which the unfelt psychic pain can be dramatized and eventually relieved' (Sidoli 2000: 97). Many patients present in the consulting-room because the dissociative defence is beginning to crumble, they find themselves on the verge of thinking the unthinkable. They reach out for help on the threshold of allowing such split-off psychic pain into mind. Because of the way the traumatic experience is remembered in the body rather than held in mind, many clients struggle to engage with and to tolerate the psychic pain, which had at some stage been too much for them to bear that it had to be dissociated. The further struggle involved in living with uncertainty, in living with states of knowing yet not knowing causes added difficulty for both patient and therapist as they seek to engage with dissociated states of mind. These states persist because traumatic experience is held captive in implicit memory and has not yet become part of autobiographical memory, accessible at will.

Nijenhuis and van der Hart (1999) define dissociative defence mechanisms as primary if the individual is distanced from the experience which is available only in flashbacks, secondary if the different aspects of experience become dissociated from one another (affect from meaning for example) and tertiary if several dissociated identities with different schemas emerge during the therapy (Nijenhuis and van der Hart 1999). A patient who suffers from the complexities of severe dissociative identity disorder (DID) and in whom there are many vertical splits, with many sub-personalities, that Jung termed 'splinter psyches' (Jung 1934a: para. 203), or Chefetz (2000) refers to as alternative subjectivities, does not have a coherent inner core that would allow her or him to move seamlessly between the different aspects of personality which emerge in different contexts.

Nijenhuis et al. (2004) have explored the way in which dissociation involves the maintenance of an effective defensive system on the one hand alongside an entirely separate system geared to managing the ordinary events of a daily life on the other. The contribution that such a split makes towards survival is seen nowhere more plainly than in the dilemma of the child who, abused by a relative at night, must sit down at breakfast with him/her the next morning as if nothing untoward had occurred. The researchers develop Myers' (1940) concept of primary structural dissociation as a division 'between the "apparently normal" personality and the "emotional" personality' (Nijenhuis et al. 2004: 2). They understand the emotional personality, which they term the EP, to be 'stuck in the traumatic experience that persistently fails to become a narrative memory of the trauma' (Nijenhuis et al. 2004: 2). They understand the apparently normal personality (ANP) to be characterized by 'avoidance of the traumatic memories, detachment, numbing, and partial or complete amnesia' (Nijenhuis et al. 2004: 2). They argue that each displays a different psychobiological response to trauma memories, which includes a different sense of self.

They point out the particular difficulty that is presented when trauma is experienced in the early years where the brain is still insufficiently developed for an integrated sense of self to have emerged. They make clear that 'the relatively low integrative level of young children can be related to the fact that brain regions that have major integrative functions, such as the prefrontal cortices and the hippocampus, have not yet fully matured' (Nijenhuis et al. 2004: 16). They also point out that the integrative capacity of children is also limited by the quality of parenting they receive. The experience of trauma will further impair their capacity to develop in an integrated way. They conclude that treatment must be geared to 'integration of feared mental contents in ways that are adapted to the current integrative capacity of the patient' (Nijenhuis et al. 2004: 21).

In both children and adults, knowledge of the trauma often intrudes in the form of repetitive thoughts, a repetitive dream or repetitive play. Terr (1991) stresses that such repetitive activities are likely to indicate experience of unresolved trauma. The clinical material that follows here illustrates something of the complexity of working with a child who has suffered early relational trauma.

The description given by a colleague of the play of a young boy in his therapy session explicated the nature of the traumatic defence more clearly than I could ever hope to do, so I shall let his play explain in the brief extract that will be given.

Jay

Miranda Davies (2002), a Jungian child analyst, saw a 13-year-old boy, Jay, who both physically and psychologically presented as a much younger child. The boy painted a graphic picture of the defences occasioned by trauma as for many sessions he played and replayed a football game with toy wild animals. His analyst experienced dissociation in the form of mindless boredom at the endless repetition and an inability to think about the meaning of the play. I was struck by the neuropsychobiological significance underlying the symbolism of the figures Jay had chosen; in conversation his analyst and I were able to explore the significance of the football game in a way that allowed meaning making to occur. On the wing was the cheetah, named by Jay after a player called 'Rush' because he could run as fast as the wind to get out of danger (flight). As forwards were a pig and a bull, named by the child after English footballers notoriously associated with aggression (fight). If all else failed the large polar bear from the land of ice occupied the goal (freeze). Hope, but also the internal struggle, was symbolized by the little kangaroo. He could break all the rules, carry the ball and run where he liked. I understood these images as attempts of the mind to represent those experiences that had remained encapsulated in the emotional brain, as yet not available to conscious mind, not yet stored in explicit memory but rather held in implicit memory. Through this metaphorical play he sought to begin to explore his defences yet in such a way that for his analyst they remained out of mind.

Terr (1991) writes of the monotonous repetitive play that is the product of traumatic experience and the difficulty that the analyst experiences in helping the child to make the links that enable the processing of the experience, thus allowing the child to move from the concrete to the symbolic. This is often because the first counter-transferential response in the therapist is a dissociative one. Davies (2002) has written more fully about this child in the *Journal of*

Analytical Psychology. I want to explore one aspect of Jay's way of being in the consulting-room, that is his play.

In his first session he lined all the toy animals from his box up, first in order of height and then of weight, clearly expressing anxiety about the hospital visits he experienced as a result of his failure to grow. Davies experienced tedium and a wiping out of her mind. Jay had found a way to play out his anxiety while keeping it out of mind for himself and his therapist. Yet he enabled his therapist to know what that felt like, albeit unconsciously. Through her reflection on her countertransference, she was able to realize something of what this defence felt like for Jay.

Davies explains that at the time of his therapy, her patients' boxes of toys were kept in a locked cupboard in her room. Usually she had no difficulty remembering to get the right box out for each child so it was with dismay that at the beginning of his fourth session she noticed she had accidentally put out another child's box. Jay seemingly shrugged the incident off and turned to the animals. Davies writes:

> He put all the black animals on one side and the white animals on the other side and played chess with them. They were turned into ciphers to be manipulated according to the rules of the game, with no animal liveliness and no trace of activity that would express feelings on Jay's behalf about the experience of being confused with another child. Following this incident, each week the animals were lined up in alphabetical order, which I found a tedious exercise. Occasionally he tossed up and dropped on my desk a pair of piglets as if they were a pair of dice. He had marked them with a felt pen on their sides, back and belly so that the score of the throw could be calculated.
>
> (Davies 2002: 427)

Davies recognized the links between Jay's play and an inner world that was derived from an infancy spent in care before adoption at 22 months old. His nursery had not assigned individual carers to the babies but rather had looked after them on a random, whoever happens to be at hand basis. By the time he was adopted at 22 months the critical period of brain development in relation to a caring mother had passed. However, it seems to me that Jay in his repetitive play was trusting his therapist enough to reveal the bare bones of his trauma. It may be that he was impelled from within to repetitive play and could do no other. However, the link Davies made to her own momentary failure to relate to Jay as an individual, when she got out the wrong toy-box, gives me hope that he was able to bring his anger at such treatment, both then and from his earlier experience, to her through the play. Indeed she concludes that 'he could convey meaning in a way that seems astonishing in a child with such early and severe deprivation' (Davies 2002: 427). Davies understood her failure to put out the right box as acting in the countertransference, that at an unconscious level Jay was enabling her to understand what it felt like to be cared for as an object rather than an individual.

Davies goes on to explore this in terms of projective identification and internal working models. I find myself thinking of an archetypal longing for a mother–child relationship, an experience of mother that enabled this child to continue to reach out to his therapist, albeit through the most painful of mediums for both, that is repetitive trauma-related play. Davies noted that in the football game Jay's archetypal fantasy of the baby kangaroo who could take a free kick and score from the other end of the field, who could run faster than all the other players, and who did not even need other players to back him up, was an amazingly accurate depiction of

> the defensive, do-it-yourself, heroic psychology of the deprived infant, who has not got the emotional resources to acknowledge his dependency on a mother figure but sustains himself with the omnipotent fantasy that he can overcome all odds and supply his own needs by his own efforts.
>
> (Davies 2002: 431)

Jay, 13 years old, but looking much younger, at the beginning of therapy, was seeking to engage with the struggles appropriate to adolescence but from the intra-psychic world of a deprived infant. He was failing academically at school and his behaviour was becoming increasingly unacceptable. Indeed the baby kangaroo's tendency to break all the rules warns that this will be the case. Davies comments:

I found the play to be defensive and self-compensatory, cutting him off from reality and building a massive protective wall around the frightened, vulnerable, desperately wounded infant at the core of his personality.

(Davies 2002: 431)

Can treatment of such early trauma work? We have a saying in England that 'the proof of the pudding is in the eating'. His school reported that by the end of his therapy he was producing four times as much written work and the behavioural difficulties experienced in school before the therapy began had ceased. He was able to move successfully into ordinary state schooling for the last phase of his education. His therapist would have liked to work longer with Jay, understanding the deep-seated tentacles that trauma inserts into personality development. Here she encountered one of the difficulties that will be familiar to all who work with parents and children, that is, the family's desire to end therapy as soon as something approaching normality is achieved.

Integration

Schore (in press) has cautioned against the lop-sidedness of analytic theory that has been for too long left brain dominated, using the left brain tool of interpretation as the main agent of change. Verbal, cognitive left brain communication between patient and analyst is not on its own sufficient cure for right brain, affective dissociative distress. For our dissociative patients it is important that the analyst engage the right brain in an empathic mode of working towards relational change but while, crucially, remaining able to think.

Emergent self-experience

In the following process material from sessions with an adult patient, Philip, I seek to illustrate ways of working in the consulting-room to modify the effects of traumatic early experience that have been compounded by later trauma. R. Moulds suggests that the suffering and the uncried tears of the trauma patient are like a huge weight of water, pent up behind a dam. The dam is like the dissociative barrier, which protects against the overwhelming stimulus. She cautions the analyst:

> Don't try to break the dam down, that would lead to destruction and devastation because of the sudden overwhelming flood of emotion. What is necessary is a tap in the dam wall that can be turned on just a little so the water can trickle away, a little at a time. That way the patient's grief and distress can be managed safely.
>
> (R. Moulds, unpublished communication, 2001)

Philip

Managing and modifying distress

Philip was a first child; his father was away abroad for most of the pregnancy and the first six months of his son's life. Philip felt that he never liked him. His mother was an anxious woman, given to illness, who found it difficult to meet the needs of her newborn son. Her own experience of mothering had been inadequate. She resorted to a strict schedule of care for her son in order to 'get it right' and to avoid the intense ambivalence she actually felt towards this child. In response to a request from her daughter-in-law about how best to care for her first child, she told her of 'sitting on the stairs, listening to Philip crying more and more desperately, looking at my watch and waiting for it to be the correct time to pick him up for his feed'. In the sessions I soon became aware of how frightened Philip was of any sense of being controlled, how difficult sticking to time and the analytic frame was for him, how difficult it was to lie down on the couch (he felt he would not be able to breathe properly and preferred to half lie, half sit). Soon I met his cold, internal controlling mother, hidden behind a seemingly compliant and adaptive self. Philip, who felt he could not bear to be controlled, sought to control me, and to undermine the control exerted by the analytic frame, by arriving late and by constant requests to change the time or the day of sessions.

Philip felt that he had become a solitary child who was treated as an object to be cared for rather than a person. He was sent away to strangers at 3 years old when his sister was to be born and to boarding school at 10 years old when his brother arrived. Philip remembers that his father told him, 'It's because you're so difficult'. His mother warned him that the other boys would bully him when he started at boarding school but that he must not make a fuss as it always happened. When Philip had been in therapy for some time, his mother died. Philip returned to his old home for the funeral and bumped into an old classmate who said, 'How are you? I had to have counselling because of the cruel way we bullied you at school'. Philip felt sick and thought he would faint as with a rush the memory of the bullying began to return. He felt that until that moment he had managed to keep it almost entirely out of mind; however, it soon became clear how accurately his body had always remembered. This will become clear in the process recording that follows.

The incident that Philip focused on most and which became the most frightening for him took place in the dormitory that he shared with fifteen other 10–12-year-old boys. His mattress was put on the floor and he was forced to lie down on it. Another mattress was put on top of him. His memory is that the bully in charge made him do this and then made all the other children climb on top of the other mattress and jump up and down. Philip felt that the bell rescued him just when another bigger bully had come into the room and asked, 'What's HE done now?' His earliest, baby experience of lying on his back, helpless and experiencing an acute level of distress, then encountering a mother who arrived in much the same way as the bully, is echoed poignantly in his account of the school experience. Without the confirming memory of the schoolmate who brought this back to mind for my patient, such a memory might have been regarded as 'false', and the patient in danger of being abused yet again on the couch.

In the following extract Philip describes the beginnings of his dissociation of this incident and then in the session the dissociation begins to dissolve and together we try to become more in touch, in a bearable amount, with the terror and pain of his 10-year-old child self.

P: (*speaking in a child-like voice, very different from that of the cultured middle-aged man who is my patient*) You had to do what they said. You couldn't not. (*Philip was looking frightened, his eyes became restless and his hands began to clench and unclench convulsively, he rubbed his upper arms.)*

M: How did that feel?

P: It was an awful feeling, and you know that other boy, well he was a bully too and he said, 'What's HE done?'

M: That must have been very frightening, if he was a bully too and he was a bigger boy.

P: *(suddenly talking brightly now but in a rather clipped way)* Yes and the bell and you had to wipe your face, wipe it all off and go to lessons.

I was caught in the feeling of the child who was trying desperately to dissociate, to change from one world to another and the sheer effort that this would require emotionally. I was shifting with him to remain in the empathic dance. The need here was for that fine balance that retains the empathy but nevertheless begins to undo the dissociation. This process becomes possible because in the therapist both experiences are held together.

M: That must have been really difficult?

P: *(cheerily)* Oh no I liked the lessons, asking questions and all that.

(I was quiet, still emotionally aware of the child who had suffered in the dormitory.)

P: *(began to speak quietly and in a wondering sort of way, turning to look into my eyes as he spoke)* Do you know I think I just split it all off, while we had lessons I just forgot and enjoyed them.

M: And after? *(My tone sought to express the empathic, right brain limbic way of working we all use so frequently, while the question sought to continue the undoing of the dissociation.)*

P: I used to try and hide. You know one of the worst things was you couldn't tell anyone at school. There was no one to tell and if you had you would get bullied worse.

M: And you couldn't tell at home because your mother had warned you to expect to be bullied at school.

(Philip told the bullying incident again but with less fear, keeping eye contact with me the whole time he was telling it.)

M: How did it feel?

P: *(speaking very quietly after a long pause)* Like unimaginable pain.

(We were both silent for a while holding in mind the boy, his sadness and his pain.)

P: I could have died.

M: *(thinking of Philip's fear of not being able to breathe)* You mean you might have suffocated?

P: *(Seeming not to hear what I said)* I could have died. I could have. People die from crush injuries. *(Suddenly there was a look of absolute horror on his face and I felt as if we were both back there for a moment with the mattress on top of us, and numerous children bouncing up and down on it.)* People die from crush injuries.

Philip looked down at his body and his arms as if he were seeing them anew. It came to mind that this patient had suffered from arthritis at a much earlier age than is usual. I said quietly, 'Your body remembers'. Somehow the moment moved on and Philip began to speak of his work with vulnerable children. He suddenly recalled a judge saying to him, 'Some abuse it would be impossible for a child to imagine'. There was a chill in the room. Philip recalled that it was his old classmate, being unable to forget the horror of what the boys had done, who had enabled Philip to remember the abuse he had suffered at school. In the session Philip clearly recalled, indeed re-experienced the hostile faces of the children around him. When he retold the story it was apparent that he paused several times and looked long at my face as if he was processing the difference and through that cortical processing, a process which engaged both hemispheres of his brain. He gradually became able to modify the effects of terror as it was represented to him by his amygdaloidal response to hostile faces.

Hariri et al. (2000) have been able to show that when presented with angry or fearful faces activation in higher cortical areas can inhibit amygdala response to the stimuli that would otherwise drive the fear response (Hariri et al. 2000, cited in Canli 2004: 1113–14). Canli also cites a further study by Ochsner et al. (2002) who scanned subjects as they appraised highly negative images. They were also able to demonstrate that increased cortical activity 'modulated activity in other regions associated with emotion processing' (Canli 2004: 1115).

At the beginning of therapy the greatest need may be for

containment, with the therapist as the container of uncontainable affect, of unbearable experience. The therapist is also the one who can process the rapidly changing dynamics of the transference and countertransference in order that what feels like 'now' may settle into 'then'. Watt discusses the nature of empathy and concludes that it *'reflects admixtures of more primitive 'affective resonance' or contagion mechanisms, melded with developmentally later-arriving emotion identification, and theory of mind/perspective taking* (Watt 2005: 185, italics in original). The former he describes as consisting of more 'unconscious, automatic imitation' [working] on much faster time-scales' (Watt 2005: 203). Thus he might be said to propose a top-down and bottom-up theory of empathy. Once the empathic relationship is established, a need for meaning making will develop, for naming that which was previously known only in the body, unavailable to the mind. Sidoli (2000) gives a sensitive account of her approach to work with such patients. I want to give a flavour of her approach here as it is very much in keeping with my own.

> The analyst must pay a great deal of attention to the subliminal messages conveyed by the body and much less attention to the verbal, factual report. The unintegrated emotional fragments are located in the body. Thus one must listen with a 'third ear' and observe with a 'third eye' . . . my countertransference with these patients is rooted . . . most of all in my experience of observing young infants and their nonverbal way of relating . . . I have to make my way towards making the hopeless infant inside the patient trust . . . When the attachment sets in, the patient will slowly use me to make up for the mirroring experience he or she missed.
>
> (Sidoli 2000: 102)

The development of the regulation of affect within the patient brings with it the capacity to reflect, that then makes more possible the interpretative moment, in turn bringing with it the possibility of more integrated hemispheric functioning and the development of coherent narrative. For this to occur successfully interpretations must be grounded in the emotional experiencing that occurs within the therapeutic dyad rather than being merely cognitive, engaging primarily the left hemisphere. Beebe and Lachmann (2002: 17) describe this view of analytic process as 'a co-constructed interactive process'. This process of change is not only that of making unconscious conscious, as with interpretation but also relational in that the interactive experiencing within the therapeutic dyad is fundamental to the successful process of change.

Severe and sustained early relational trauma may give rise to vertical splits within the personality, experienced as alternating subjectivities. At the very least there will be the frightened, angry child, whose development was stopped by the experience of over-whelming trauma and whose emergence in the consulting-room will mark the first tentative steps towards trust. One might say that part of successful therapy will be the recognition of the three-some in the consulting-room, that is the analyst, the patient who manages the day to day more or less successfully and the inner hurt part of the patient that is often characterized as 'the traumatized child within'. The skill of the analyst is to relate to both without favouring one or the other so that the two may become more able to interact in a caring way one with the other, eventually becoming more wholly integrated into one, allowing a new experience of the self.

The questions surrounding the recall of memory and accuracy of memories that surface in the consulting-room have been widely dis-cussed, however we should also be aware of the way in which the changing of emotional memory may actually be a benign aspect of analytic work, in that the retelling (from explicit) or re-experiencing (from implicit) of memories in the presence of the therapist may lead to a modulation in the quality of the affect associated with the memory, thus modifying the memory. Most are agreed that the initial aims in therapy must be to establish a sense of safety and a capacity to self-regulate. To help the development of the capacity to self-soothe is essential to treatment of those who have been severely traumatized.

Approaches that help with the avoidance and/or management of flashbacks are fundamental. Siegel notes that 'recent studies of flashback conditions suggest an intense activation of the right hemi-sphere visual cortex and an inhibition of left hemisphere speech areas' (Siegel 2003: 15). At such moments much will depend on the calm that the therapist is able to sustain in the face of much that urges consciously and unconsciously towards just the opposite. A lowering of tone and slowing of speech, speaking in what Williams (2004) has termed 'pastel rather than primary colours' may help to counteract the responses triggered in the patient. It may be possible to help the patient to modify their experience by use of a simple phrase such as 'it was then, not now'. Cozolino (2002) suggests that this is effective because it stimulates Broca's area (that produces speech) and encourages the functioning of right and left hemispheres in a more integrated way. Siegel suggests that focusing on elements of

> both the right (imagery, bodily state, emotion, autobiographical memory) and left hemispheres (words, self-concepts, logical understanding of the cause-effect relationships among events in a linear analysis such as a narrative) enables a multidimensional representational activation [that encourages integration].
>
> (Siegel 2003: 46)

A trauma patient's early experience causes the self to retreat, hidden from the world by protective defences. The analyst who seeks to engage in work with those who dissociate may feel that they are working at the frontier, in no-man's land, at the edges of analytic understanding and practice. Lanyado (1999) stresses that until the analyst has experienced the patient's trauma in the countertransference and been genuinely shocked by it, the patient cannot begin to work on the problem of their own traumatizing behaviour. Hopkins (1986) notes that to help a patient to recover from trauma is liable to involve the therapist 'not only in sharing the pain but in suffering grave doubts about whether facing pain so starkly is necessary, and whether the self-protection of turning a blind eye may be preferable' (Hopkins 1986: 71). Solomon (1998: 237) cautions that 'the analyst will inevitably be open to suffusion by the patient's terror of the appalling potential for retraumatisation, given the inevitable failures that occur within the context of human relatedness'. Ehrlich (2003: 237) comments that when working at the frontier the analyst must be mindful that 'the frontier is also the "no-man's land" where enemies are created and come into being'. He cites Bion's comment that 'in every consulting-room there should be two rather frightened people: the patient and the psychoanalyst' (Bion 1990: 5). He suggests that 'to enable others to relate to us really and fully, that is including aggressiveness and destructiveness, what we must be capable of is not placation or masochistic surrender, or retaliatory aggression, but rather life-affirming survival' (Ehrlich 2003: 245).

Solomon explains:

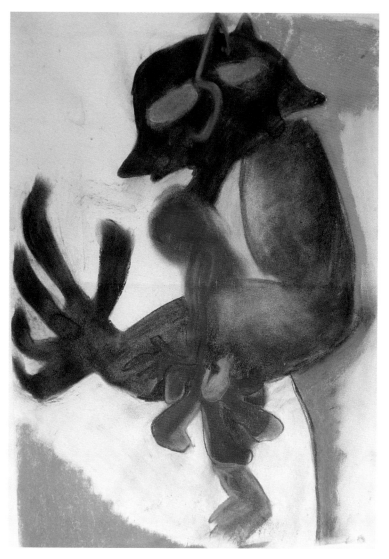

Plate 1 (Chapter 8)

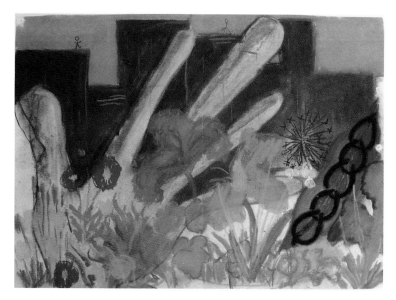

Plate 2 (Chapter 8)

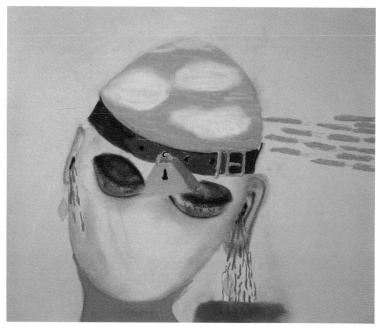

Plate 3 (Chapters 8 and 9)

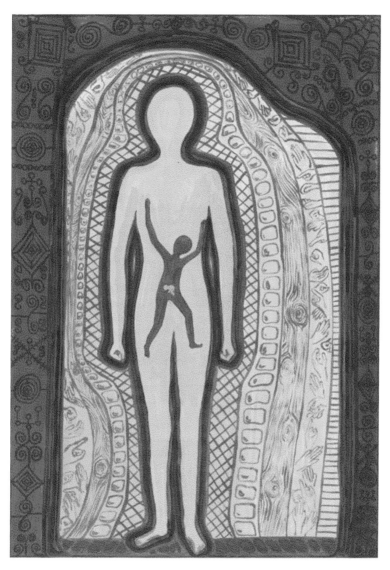

Plate 4 (Chapter 9)

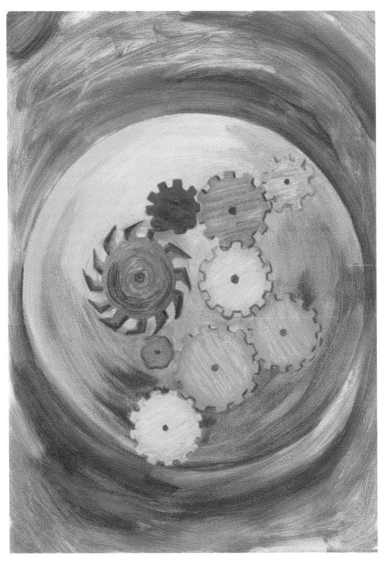

Plate 5 (Chapter 9)

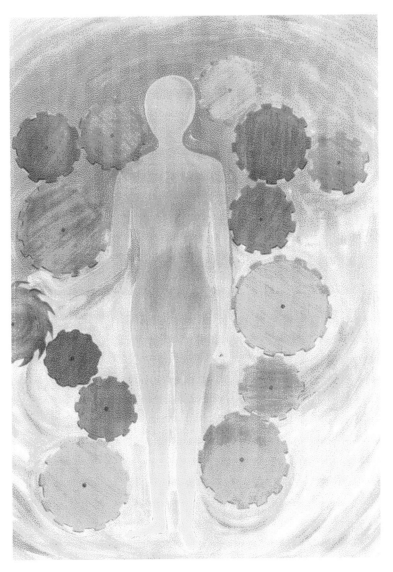

Plate 6 (Chapter 9)

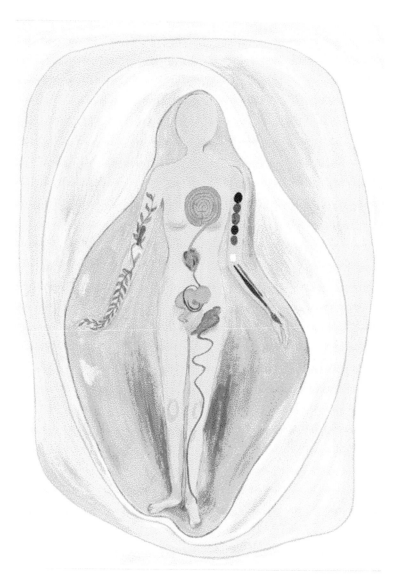

Plate 7 (Chapter 9)

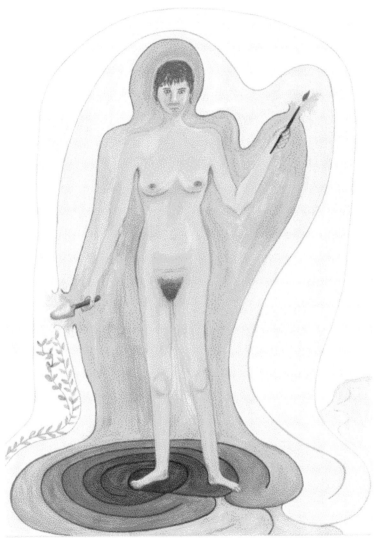

Plate 8 (Chapter 9)

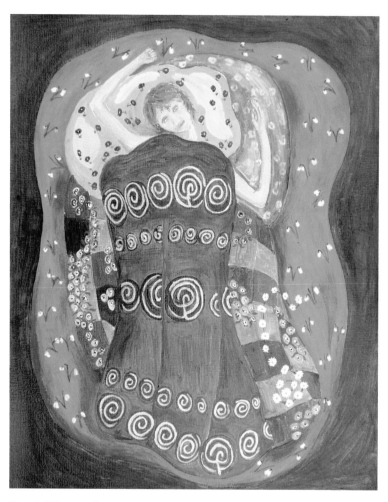

Plate 9 (Chapter 9)

Because the substantive reality of the existence of the patient's self was eschewed by their important others, the self was experienced as extremely poisonous to the self, or as a bizarre object that was liable to appropriate a part of the self and render it alien or mad.

(Solomon 2004: 644)

She suggests that both empathic understanding and focused thinking are vital components in processing what might otherwise be experienced as unbearably toxic and repelling (Solomon 2004: 650).

Bromberg suggests that one aim of analytic work is to allow such patients to 'experience a spontaneous overflow of powerful feelings as safe rather than fearsome and shame ridden' (Bromberg 2003: 708). He concludes that what is needed in order to do this is 'a "safe-enough" interpersonal environment' (Bromberg 2003: 708). Ehrlich (2003) suggests that yesterday's danger zone may become today's sphere of creative innovation; indeed it may be so with the consulting-room and the analytic dyad, but not without the capacity for repair and for reconciliation. It is often just that experience of rupture, repair and reconciliation that builds new confidence in the relationship and that enables our dissociative patients gradually to drop the defence that, although originally life-saving, has become life-denying.

Conclusion

The plasticity of the brain throughout life enables such change. The mirroring of healthy early relational experience by the therapeutic dyad permits new entities to be added to pre-existing connections in both brain-minds. Exchanges that involve putting feelings into words encourage healthy and integrated functioning of both hemispheres of the brain and are an intrinsic part of the process of coming into mind. Analytic work that encompasses relational as well as interpretive agents of change can bring about the integration and increased connectivity between and within both hemispheres of the mind-brain that lead to a change in the nature of attachment which will then permit the self to emerge more fully through the process of individuation.

Chapter 7

The adolescent brain

A new developmental stage

The adolescent brain has been described as 'a work in progress'; adolescence marks a distinct developmental stage 'second only to the neonatal period in terms of both rapid biopsychosocial growth as well as changing environmental characteristics and demands' (Schore 2003b: 297). I became particularly interested in the challenges successful negotiation of adolescence presented for young people when I worked as a school counsellor and advisory teacher for this age group. The adolescent cases that follow are composites based on the experience that I gained through working in an educational setting with many adolescents whose difficulties manifested themselves in problems with school attendance. My interest has been sustained by the number of young and not so young adults that I have seen in whom adolescent states of mind predominate, particularly at the beginning of therapy. Astor (1988: 70–1) traces the development of analytic thought about adolescent states of mind in adult patients in the work of Meltzer (1973), Bion (1977) and Fordham (1985).

Michael Fordham, in conversation with Astor, emphasized the need to be aware of the child in the adult not merely as symbolic but also as 'the child in the adult as a body . . . a reference to the bodily relation of the child to its mother' (Astor 2005: 13). Sidoli (2000) has developed Fordham's insight concerning the bodily relation to the mother in her writing with her emphasis on the need for the therapist to consider what the patient's body might be communicating. The new understanding we have of the brain focuses attention on the unitary nature of the mind-brain-body being. The particular qualities of adolescence require us to adopt a similar perspective in consideration of adolescent patients and adolescent states of mind in adult patients.

In adolescence there is a second wave of nerve cell production followed by neural pruning; the 'use it or lose it' principle is seen at work for the second time paralleling the process of development that occurs in the first 18 months of life. Just as the earlier stage coincides with the beginnings of an awareness of others and the development of what has been termed 'the neural substrate of shame', so this stage, when the capacity for reasoning and judgement begins to gradually mature, takes place when the young person begins to separate from their parents and to engage more with the outside world. The adolescent slowly begins to be able to be more aware of the effects of actions on others and to be able to inhibit impulsive behaviours. As in the earlier stage the limbic areas (concerned with emotional responses) mature earlier than the frontal lobes (concerned with judgement and reasoning). However, just as in the earlier stage, development is uneven with emotional development outpacing executive control; it is out of this unevenness of development that much of the difficulty experienced in adolescence arises.

Brain changes

The decade of the brain has allowed the first detailed age-related studies of the changes in the volume of grey and white matter in both childhood and adolescence. In adolescence there is a marked growth spurt in grey matter that is followed by what appears to be an extensive pruning process; however, the amount of myelinated neurons, those with axons clothed in myelin, the white matter that insulates and therefore makes them effective transmitters, increases at this stage. A gain in the amount of myelinated neurons leads to faster and more effective communication within the brain. While acknowledging recent advances in our ability 'to relate structural and functional maturation of the adolescent brain to that of the adolescent's behaviour' (Paus 2005: 60), Paus notes that while there is growing agreement that there is a continuous increase throughout adolescence in the amount of white matter, science is not yet able to distinguish definitively whether grey matter is actually lost or whether it is rather a case of those cells becoming coated (Paus 2005: 60). If it is the latter, the process probably reflects the increasing neural connectivity in the brain that results from the enriched environmental interactions that are part of the fuller life experience of the teenager.

Much is still to be explored, for example Siegel observes that the way in which 'genetically coded information interacts with environmental and interactive elements to determine the nature of this important adolescent pruning period is open to future investigation' (Siegel 2003: 11). The nature/nurture debate continues: Paus observes that 'it is equally probable that a (pre-existing) variation in structure could affect performance or that a repeated engagement of a given circuit could change brain morphology' (Paus 2005: 63). Several studies have looked at the changes in the adolescent brain over time. Gogtay et al. (2004) used biennial MRI scans to track the changes in the grey matter development between the ages of 4 and 21 in a group of 13 healthy children and noted the pattern of the wave of brain changes, observing that the frontal lobes mature last (Gogtay et al. 2004: 8176). Paus et al. (1999), in a study of 111 children, were able to demonstrate age-related increases in white matter density in fibre tracts, providing evidence for a gradual maturation of fibre pathways thought to be involved in speech and motor function (Paus et al. 1999: 1908). Paus emphasizes that such use of structural MRI (for example to demonstrate that neuronal tracts connecting different regions of the brain thicken as they become coated with the protective sheath of myelin) has opened up 'unprecedented opportunities for studying the neural substrates [of development]' (Paus 2005: 60).

In 1998 Yurgelun-Todd noted the difference between responses to pictures of fearful faces between adolescents and adults. In both adults and adolescents the amygdala was responsive; in the adults, the prefrontal cortex was also activated but significantly not in the adolescents (Yurgelun-Todd 1998, cited in Schore 2003b: 174). Thus, as in childhood, the limbic area matures before the frontal cortex meaning that emotional states, including desire, may dominate and prove difficult for the young adolescent to control. Again the adolescent brain may be understood as 'a work in progress'; in this case the inhibition of emotional response by the prefrontal cortex is as yet incomplete. This is significant for the understanding that the parent and therapists must bring to interactions with this age group. It also means that analysis and therapy must as always be rooted in the relational, that the therapist must seek to work associatively, encouraging connectivity, and that left brain, interpretational interventions should be used to underpin this rather than be the sole approach used for young people of this age group.

The effects of trauma

Relational trauma in both early years and in adolescence affects healthy brain development. Unresolved conflicts from early years challenge the adolescent who is struggling to develop an adequate sense of identity, a sense of self as separate yet in healthy relation to others. Bronstein (2004) observes that the changes experienced in adolescence and their accompanying anxieties 'evoke again the intense experiences and anxieties of early infancy. Such experiences . . . now reawaken in a radically new setting that of a sexually mature body' (Bronstein 2004: 23). For children who have experienced early relational trauma and who already have as a result excessively pruned cortical subcortical circuits, this stage of life can be overwhelming. Further pruning of these already excessively pruned circuits leads to inability to develop or sustain frontal lobe regulation. The resultant inability to self-regulate reveals itself in impulsive, sometimes aggressive or fearful amygdala-driven behaviours. Father-hunger and father-thirst originating at toddler stage (see Chapter 3) may now turn to rage, despair and finally to dissociative reactions if father still remains 'absent' as the teenager struggles with the return of similar developmental pressures. In 2004 researchers showed that there was a higher risk of adolescent males going to prison if they came from homes where there was an absent father. However, the group who faced the highest risk were those from stepfamilies, including father-stepmother families (Harper and McLanahan 2004: 369).

Putnam (1997), in his discussion of dissociative responses to trauma in children and adolescents, stresses that abuse whether physical, psychological or sexual along with neglect is implicated in the kinds of difficulties that arise in adolescence. He particularly notes the high correlation with the incidence of self-harm, substance abuse and somatisation, and the lack of significant evidence for genetic contributions to pathological dissociation. He notes that 'core dissociative features are found in common across widely divergent cultures' (Putnam 1997: 197). In 2004 researchers reported that a large-scale study of 1696 young people drawn from the United States, China, Korea and the Czech Republic revealed considerable similarity in the part played by family factors in adolescent depressive symptomatology and problem behaviours (Dmitrieva et al. 2004). In a substantial study Teicher (2000) has linked sexual abuse to disturbances of the healthy development of the limbic system (similar to that experienced by patients with temporal lobe epilepsy), and of the corpus callosum (the main information highway between the left and right hemispheres), and of the healthy functioning of the left hemisphere. Some researchers, including Teicher (2000), are pessimistic about the possibility of change for those so affected. However, many others such as Cozolino, LeDoux, Pally, Perry and van der Kolk argue that change is possible. Pally (2000) points out that 'since it is known that consciously attending to and verbalising something can enhance cortical activation . . . treatments such as analysis . . . take advantage of cortical plasticity, to modulate deeply engrained emotional responses' (Pally 2000: 15). Adolescence is generally agreed to encompass three stages that embrace early teens, mid-teens and late teens into early twenties.

Early adolescence

Early adolescence is generally held to be the period in the early teen or even pre-teen years when the young person's body begins to change and to mature in ways that may seem strange to the 'child' who inhabits it. This is particularly true for the child whose experience in infancy and childhood has been less than adequate, the only memory of which may be held in the very body that begins to experience strange new sensations. These sensations may be experienced as disturbing in new and old ways. This is especially so in the case of children who have experienced physical trauma (for example illness, hospitalization and invasive procedures) or physical or sexual abuse in early childhood. An adolescent may 'experience his/her body as "bad" or "wrong", containing all the rejected unlovable aspects of him/herself' (Bronstein 2004: 27). Eating disorders, self-harming, cutting and suicidal behaviours may emerge at this stage. Dissociation as a defence may become part of the clinical picture, particularly if dissociative patterns have developed in childhood as strategies for coping with unduly stressful experience. As one's sense of self arises out of bodily experience so the young person may begin to experience uncertainty about just who he or she is. Astor (1988) describes the way in which inadequate experience in early childhood leads to difficulties with the transformation of emotional, bodily experience into symbolic form that is then available to be thought about (Astor 1988: 71). Trauma at this stage can be particularly difficult to deal with, if underlying early trauma is reawakened as we shall see with Sharon.

Sharon

Sharon was the second child in a family where the first child, also a girl, had been seriously disabled from birth and was not expected to survive her first year of life. Sharon was just 13 months younger than her very disabled sibling, who survived but with frequent crises and hospitalizations. Sharon's mother was almost entirely preoccupied with her first-born child; she took little notice of the 'replacement child' who now seemed not to be wanted but rather to be an extra demand on a mother who already felt stretched to her limits. When her father came home from work his attention went first to his wife and sick child but then he would engage with Sharon so that he, rather than her mother, was her closest attachment figure. The terrible strain of disability wrought havoc with the parents' relationship. They stayed together until their elder daughter was moved into residential care at 13 years of age. Soon after, the father left, remarried and moved to a distant town. In a short space of time Sharon lost her sister and her father and was left with a distressed mother who still barely noticed her. At first she tried hard at school, unconsciously trying to find a way to please her parents and in particular to win her mother's interest and approval. She struggled, without being aware of them, with unconscious guilt feelings, first of being healthy and then of having her mother to herself. Her mother meanwhile remained frustratingly emotionally unavailable. When the full effects of adolescence struck Sharon was entirely unprepared for the onslaught. She began to act out her anger and despair, first having a string of boyfriends, going drinking and clubbing, using spirits and Ecstasy, then moving out as soon as she was 16 years old to live with a man closer to her father's age than her own, who was also a substance abuser. She began to stay away from school more and more frequently; she did not take her examinations, rather she became depressed and made several quite serious suicidal gestures. Her boyfriend moved to Scotland because of work and she went with him. She tried to start a college course but was struck by the first of what were to be many psychotic episodes necessitating in-patient treatment. Her psychiatrist attributed her state to the abuse of alcohol and drugs. It would seem that the early neglect, with its inevitable effect on brain development, followed by the loss of her father at the time of her sister's disappearance, coinciding with the developmental difficulties of puberty, heightened her vulnerability to developing drug dependence and psychotic illness.

Risk or reason?

In healthy adolescents the frontal lobes that deal with processes of reasoning and judgement are still immature, thus they are unable to look into the future and to predict consequences of their actions. This ability is thought to emerge between 15 and 18 years of age but it may be that the frontal lobes do not fully mature until a young person is 21 or even 25 years old. Restak (2001), discussing the plasticity of the adolescent brain, adds the sobering comment that 'the adolescent's choices determine the quality of his brain' (Restak 2001: 77). In the clinical vignettes you will note that sometimes it is risk-taking aggravated by the stresses in current relationships or life events that the young person is experiencing and sometimes the effect of poor or traumatic experience in early years that has resulted in a turbulent adolescence.

Plasticity permits programming

The very plasticity of the brain that we value as therapists, because it holds out the possibility of change, is sometimes the downfall of the adolescent. The brain as easily becomes programmed to patterns of abuse as to care and nurture. Carter (2000) comments:

> The brain uses a carrot and stick system to ensure that we pursue and achieve the things we need in order to survive. A stimulus from outside . . . or from the body . . . is registered by the limbic system which creates an urge which registers consciously as desire. The cortex then instructs the body to act in whatever way is necessary to achieve its desire. The activity sends messages to the limbic system which releases opioid-like neurotransmitters which raise circulating dopamine levels and create a feeling of satisfaction.

(Carter 2000: 95)

Plasticity means that development of the reward pathway that is activated in drug abuse can mean that the brain very quickly becomes wired to the overwhelming pleasure that is achieved through the use of street drugs. In adolescents who use these drugs, the brain is literally being shaped by increasing dependence on the pleasure response that comes from the 'drug associated electrochemical firing of the reward pathways of the brain' (Restak 2001: 85). Restak explains the detail of the reward pathway:

> The cascade begins when neurons in the hypothalamus release serotonin. This triggers the release of other neurotransmitters that in turn allow cells in the ventral tegmental area to release dopamine. The dopamine travels to the amygdala, the nucleus accumbens, and certain parts of the hippocampus. Along with the prefrontal cortex, these centres are involved in memory formation, explaining why visual and other cues associated with drug use can trigger intense cravings in people addicted to such substances.
>
> (Restak 2001: 84)

Thus, in the abuse of Ecstasy or cocaine, the young person's desire system is easily stimulated by the sight (outside) of the exchange of drugs or the memory (inside) of what it's like to feel high; the developed limbic system sends the message 'go for it' without inhibition from the frontal cortex which is as yet too immature to reason 'this could damage me'. The young person will go to any lengths to satisfy the desire system that has been activated. Again the frontal cortex's immaturity makes it more difficult for the adolescent to reason 'I should not be doing this', for example as he or she steals in order to support the craving. The drugs bring an overwhelming sense of satisfaction produced by the artificial introduction of serotonin in the case of Ecstasy and dopamine in the case of cocaine.

Plasticity, the power of the reward system and the as yet incomplete development of the capacity of the frontal lobes for inhibiting impulsive action means that vulnerable teenagers, who have had a poor start emotionally, are particularly at risk.

The effects of Ecstasy

MDMA, the synthetic product methylenedioxymethamphetamine, known as Ecstasy, stimulates the release of serotonin producing an euphoric high within 45 minutes, as the effects begin to wear off quite quickly the user often takes more in order to prolong the pleasurable experience. There is considerable controversy surrounding the long-term effects of Ecstasy. Research on non-humans indicates that Ecstasy acts as

> [a] selective neurotoxin, destroying the axon terminals that arise from serotonin cell bodies in the brain stem. Repeated doses of MDMA cause cumulative loss of serotonergic axon terminals in the cerebral cortex . . . studies . . . have demonstrated reduced serotonin activity in abstinent recreational Ecstasy users.
>
> (Parrott 2002: 472)

Such research would indicate that those who use Ecstasy regularly or in large quantities on a given occasion are at risk of damaging their own system for producing serotonin, resulting in long-term depression. Writing in the same issue of *The Psychologist* (September 2002) three researchers (Cole, Sumnall and Grob) argued against long-term damage; however, their views were hotly contested by Morgan (2002), Croft (2002) and Parrott (2002) in three separate responses.

Damage to brain means damage to mind

Morgan (2002: 468) suggested that his study presented 'overwhelming evidence that regular ecstasy users suffer from impulsive behaviour and deficits in verbal memory performance, and that these deficits are specifically associated with past use of ecstasy' rather than any other street drug. Croft et al. (2001) reported serotonin impairment in Ecstasy users, relative to both controls and cannabis users, and argued that this, alongside the research demonstrating decreased serotonin function in rats (Commins et al. 1987) and non-human primates (Ricaurte et al. 1988), means that the use of Ecstasy must be considered a serious threat. Parrott (2002) cites research that indicates memory deficits resulting from the use of Ecstasy (Zakanis and Young 2001) and notes that further research has shown these deficits to be greater in those who are heavy rather than light users of the substance (Fox et al. 2001a, 2001b) and notes that Ecstasy users report significantly higher depression and less sociability than non-users. He concludes that the notion that these deficits are imaginary as hypothesized by Cole et al. (2002) is 'negated by the brain scan literature, the consistency of human functional deficits, and the extensive animal data' (Parrott 2002: 473).

Middle adolescence

Brafman (2004: 46) describes the mid-teen period as the years when 'youngsters have to fumble their way through disentangling the values of their earlier life that they wish to continue to adopt from those they wish to discard'. He notes the 'unconscious (and sometimes conscious) ambivalence about the disengagement' (Brafman 2004: 46). As young people struggle with ambivalent feelings about parents and experience a fluctuating need to be close and to separate, experience which is challenging in this area can be particularly difficult to manage. Traumatic experience can impact adversely on the young person's attempts to negotiate this stage of development.

Charlie

The experience of Charlie demonstrates the added risk to which a young person is exposed if they have to deal with repeated trauma at this vulnerable stage in the attainment of maturity and independence. Charlie was the victim of a road traffic accident when he was almost 15 years old. Charlie and two friends had left his parents, who were at a party at their neighbours' house, to walk the short distance home so that they could go and listen to some music. As they walked along a motor-bike careered off the road, mounted the pavement and hit Charlie. According to the driver, who stopped and called an ambulance, Charlie did not lose consciousness and he was conscious when the paramedics arrived. However, Charlie remembered nothing of the incident from beginning the walk home to coming round in hospital in severe pain with his mother at his bedside.

Initially it seemed that Charlie was the victim of this single horrifying event. Gradually it became clear that the young Charlie had experienced not one but three frightening events that emphasized to him his helplessness and lack of ability to keep safe. A year or so before his own accident, the whole family had been involved in a motorway crash, all were unhurt but it compounded his later fright. As a young child he had had emergency in-patient treatment for a severe infection. Thus when he found himself in hospital with a badly broken pelvis, the result of the accident with the motor-bike, earlier layers of distress were reactivated.

When Charlie emerged from hospital and returned to school he had built a protective wall of denial around his experiences. He avoided speaking about any aspect of the accident to anyone, but he suffered from frightening dreams at night and intrusive thoughts by day. He began to seek ways of putting the trauma out of mind, of keeping the terror at bay. Over the next eighteen months he began to 'bunk off' single lessons, then half days. When he found that he 'got away with it', the absence escalated until he began to miss whole days of school. He found smoking cannabis gave some relief and an escape from unbearable thoughts. He drank and partied, sometimes using Ecstasy. He felt himself to be at risk but could not control it. His parents were concerned, hoped it was 'just a phase' and found 'No' only exacerbated the situation. They wisely sought other ways to help their son. His father thought that maybe some therapy would help and he persuaded Charlie to come to see me.

Time had become skewed for Charlie as the trauma of his accident threw shadows both backward and forward. Charlie felt that he was closest to his father and his younger brother was closest to his mother. Sometimes he was able to be aware of his parents' closeness to him, at other times he spoke of feeling always alone and close to no one. I became aware of his fears that there was no one to keep him safe, that sometimes he felt as if it had been that way forever. Gradually he came to understand that this second layer of feeling about his parents was part of the shadow cast by the accident, and the earlier difficult experience he had had in hospital as a very small child. Indeed Charlie, like so many trauma victims (Terr 1991: 13–14), was unable to imagine a safe future. It felt that the next accident or disaster was lurking just around the corner. In therapy he struggled with the experience of hospital and what he felt was his mother's failure to tell the nurses of his need for better pain control. This perception lasted over many therapy sessions until suddenly he became able to realize that the accident, not his mother, was responsible for his pain. However, once again he had to confront knowledge of utter helplessness and frightening feelings concerning the random element of chance in life, a difficult experience for a boy just entering adolescence with his fears and longings concerning separateness, autonomy and the ability to function independently.

After we had been meeting for about six months, Charlie and his family went abroad on a skiing holiday. It was rare for the family to be able to spend time together and it helped to 'settle' Charlie. He began to attend school more regularly. He studied hard and did quite well in spite of the amount of school he had missed over the years. He decided to stay on in the sixth form for an extra year to get results that would enable him to enter college, whereas previously he had not felt able to do so. While he gradually became free of his daily playbacks of the trauma his underlying anxieties about a certain future remained. However, his parents reported that the lively boy with a teasing sense of humour that everyone knew before the accident was gradually beginning to re-emerge from time to time. With his experience of catastrophe he could not always sustain this; a sense of going safely and strongly into the world had somehow become elusive. He felt the need to sleep a lot; study seemed overwhelming at times, and the thought of the future that he was told he should study for, intangible. Further progress came with the advent of a steady girlfriend, a relationship that seemed overall to be supportive. About this time I became unwell and a two-week school holiday break became four. This was very hard for Charlie. He could not tolerate the thought of weakness or helplessness in me, it felt far too scary. He returned with difficulty after the break, often it seemed he 'accidentally' arranged to be at extra Maths lessons or to be committed to school sports events at times that coincided with the therapy. He chose to end his therapy at the end of the school year as he was mostly symptom free and his parents began to feel he was his old self again. He continued to drink quite freely at weekends but no longer smoked cannabis or used Ecstasy. His difficulty with work and need for sleep may well have been at least in part the aftermath of the substance abuse to which he had turned in an effort to keep the trauma at bay, in the period before he came into therapy. His ability to gain control over his impulsive behaviour had much to do with the quality of parenting he received at the time and the use he was able to make of me in the therapy.

Traditionally analysts have linked the capacity to relate to the outside world to the relation with the father. While Stern (1985) has noted the unconscious technique of purposeful misattunement used first by the mother and then by other close care-givers in the second year of life, analysts have also emphasized the father's role as the bridge to the outside world at this time. In adolescence the need for a bridge to the outside world becomes even more apparent and the problems for teenagers who have maintained too close a tie to the mother are well documented. Charlie and another teenager, each of whom I saw once a week for over a year, caused me to think carefully about the links between the maturing brain and the maturing mind and to consider very carefully the importance of the relation to the father in the susceptibility towards substance abuse. I surmise that as the frontal cortex, responsible for reasoning and judgement, lags behind the limbic system in development, the availability and internalization of a good enough parent's knowledge of when and how to say 'No' may be of crucial importance in protecting the young person from over-exposure to uncontrolled, impulsive behaviours.

Late adolescence

This is the time when the adolescent may really begin to separate from parents, to venture forth into the world of university or of work, of digs or a shared flat. Those who remain at home may establish a degree of independence that symbolizes a new ability to separate internally, and in so doing to value the other in a new way.

Peter

Peter was referred to me by the head of his year at school. One of the brightest students in the year, Peter had been expected to do exceptionally well in the examinations that would admit him to higher education; he had been offered a provisional place at a prestigious university to read the subject of his choice. When he was 16 years old his parents had split up. He was an only child and as a young child he had felt close to both parents and very attached to his mother. At the time of the break-up it was she who had moved away with a new partner to start a new life in another city. He and his father had moved in with his paternal grandmother. At the time of the break-up, his paternal grandmother reported, he had been a sociable, sensible young man who worked very hard during the week and enjoyed going clubbing on Saturdays. Soon after his mother left he began to go out the three nights of the weekend but continued to study in the week. His father worked long hours in a low-paid job and left home early in the morning each weekday. As the examinations that would allow him entry to university drew near, his father found out that his son had ceased to attend school. It became clear that he was lying in bed all day with the curtains drawn; he'd persuaded his grandmother to say nothing about this. When asked he said that he did not feel up to getting up and going to school. After the usual gamut of hospital tests had been run and drawn a blank, he came to see me.

By the time we first met, Peter had failed to take his examinations, he was very depressed and convinced that as he felt so awful something very serious physically must be wrong with him that the doctors had missed. He agreed it might be helpful to have someone to talk to about how he felt; he spoke about how much he missed the woman French teacher who had left the school a year earlier, he felt she had understood his aspirations. I felt that she had stood in for his mother and the loss; bringing with it the failure of the illusion of mothering, meant he could no longer manage. Inevitably the transference to me was complex. He hoped that I might make the doctor understand how ill he was feeling, he was sure something was very wrong physically. Occasionally I was able to catch glimpses of the able, gutsy, independent teenager he had once been, who had loved his academic subjects, who held strong views intellectually and politically, but also a young man who had enjoyed clubbing, drinking beer and using Ecstasy. More often I met the exhausted, deeply depressed young person who just wanted to remain in bed in the dark, with the curtains drawn. Significantly he had conceived a deep dislike of his father; he felt it was his father's fault that his mother had left. In blaming his father he avoided his underlying conviction that it was his own fault that his mother had left. Although the school was some considerable distance away from his home, mostly he began to make what was for him the huge effort to attend at least on the days he had an appointment with me.

After I had seen him for six months and he was to leave school, he agreed to the family doctor's recommendation that he have a psychiatric assessment. On the recommendation of the psychiatrist, he began a course of a selective serotonin re-uptake inhibitor. Gradually his depression improved and eventually he took a job in the local supermarket. He hoped that later he might feel well enough to do a college course, hope of a first-class degree from a prestigious university had disappeared, but nevertheless he was considerably better. I have often wondered whether it was the counselling, the selective serotonin re-uptake inhibitor, or the cessation of exposure to alcohol and Ecstasy, or possibly the mixture of all three, that led to his improvement, albeit limited. I have also wondered whether, when his mother left, it was the blame that he attributed to his father, who had previously 'laid down the law' in the house, that meant that impulse driven behaviour came to dominate the life of this previously disciplined young man.

Woodhead (2005) has examined the importance of the relation to father in infancy, understanding the father as the creator of boundaries, structures and moralities, the one who separates mother and infant and who stimulates development, much as we saw with Jacques in Chapter 1. I find myself wondering about the importance of the 'good enough' father in adolescence in establishing the dominance of reason and control over impulsivity and risk. I wonder about the 'neuronal mirroring' of father that would assist in enabling the maturation of the frontal cortex to take place, without the hijacking of the reward system to the seeming delights of addiction. Delights that always prove all too transitory as the system adjusts to the abuse.

Conclusion

The plasticity and rapid change of the adolescent brain coupled with the developmental task of achieving greater separation from parents and a clear sense of self and identity make this a challenging and exciting stage of life. For the therapist there is the opportunity to capitalize on the plasticity and openness to change of the adolescent patient. The mirroring aspects of the transference are crucial at this stage as the adolescent has another developmental chance to internalize the mind of another. Schore's comment, concerning the transference in general, is therefore particularly applicable to adolescence.

> Because the transference is a reciprocal process, facially com-
> municated 'expressions of affect' that reflect changes in the
> internal state are rapidly communicated and perceptually pro-
> cessed within the affectively synchronised therapeutic dialogue.
> (Schore 2003b: 51)

Schore emphasizes that resonance is one of the more significant factors determining synchronization of processes within the whole brain and goes on to argue that it is affective resonance of right brain states in the analytic dyad as well as in the nursing couple that will enable change. I think the intensity of the encounter with the adolescents or those adults in whom adolescent states of mind pre-dominate, who are engaged in finding themselves through their rela-tion to others, enables the therapist to make very effective use of the underlying brain processes of resonance and synchronization to establish the right brain-based affective empathy that will carry the adolescent through the more difficult moments in the therapy. However, this can be effective only if the analyst also adequately recognizes and acknowledges existence of these states alongside the adolescent's search for separateness and identity.

This can be particularly difficult with adolescents who may use the defences aptly described by Sidoli (2000), writing of her work with one suicidal young man that 'he wore the conversational per-sona as a mask and wanted to make me and everyone else believe that, indeed, he was all right' (Sidoli 2000: 47). In her account of this work she emphasizes the importance of the bodily counter-transference in the analyst's ability to understand 'the untrans-formed early infantile experiences which have not been made sense of, primarily by the mother, in the dyadic relationship', in order to assist the young person in the process of 'naming the nameless' (Sidoli 2000: 47). Bovensiepen (2002) emphasizes the importance of the process of developing a symbolic space in work with children and adolescents. He believes this arises from 'the matrix of the transference/countertransference . . . which, like the early mother–child relationship, can lead to a transformation of emotional experience in a dyadic relationship' (Bovensiepen 2002: 252). Thus while the importance of adolescence is often emphasized in terms of the revisiting of oedipal experience, for many troubled adolescents, or adults troubled by predominantly adolescent states of mind, therapy will mean revisiting much earlier developmental experience that was not successfully negotiated in the earliest relation to the primary care-giver. Culbert-Koehn (1997), writing about regressive states in adult patients, identifies the feelings of 'smallness, helplessness and shame, when dependency on the analyst is exposed' (Culbert-Koehn 1997: 102). These kinds of feelings are particularly difficult for the adolescent state of mind to bear and need careful management. Feldman (2004) emphasizes the severe and early damage to the symbolic function that was revealed in his analytic work with a bulimic patient in late adolescence; he stresses the critical need 'to create a safe space where the emotional reactions to the early infant/mother relationship could be experienced and worked through in the analytical interaction' (Feldman 2004: 309). Sensitive work is clearly required, with an ability to work at the earliest levels while respecting and supporting the emergent adult self, whether in the adolescent, or out of the adolescent state of mind that may predominate in an adult patient. I suggest that right brained to right brained affective synchrony is the key to successful negotiation of these challenges.

Chapter 8

The dreaming mind-brain

> Dreams do not deceive, they do not lie, they do not distort or disguise, but naively announce what they are and what they mean . . . they are invariably seeking to express something that the ego does not know and does not understand.
>
> (Jung 1946: para. 189)

The American writer, Lucy Daniels, describes rather evocatively what her dreams mean for her. She comments:

> Dreams have served my creative purpose both as alarm clocks and teddy bears. They wake me to new awareness of the shackles left from my unfortunate childhood [and] . . . by continually providing evidence of my current psychological landscape, they give me the information and courage to advance both consciously and unconsciously.
>
> (Daniels 2000: 10)

In this chapter I examine insights from contemporary neuroscience concerning the nature of the dreaming process and seek to demonstrate the way in which the relevance of Jung's basic premise that dreams reveal rather than disguise the emotional concerns of the dreamer is supported by research in this field. My central thesis is that the dreaming mind-brain uses vivid visual imagery to process emotional states of mind, that are implicit, not yet available to consciousness, which seek to emerge, through the vehicle of the dream, into consciousness where they may be thought about. Further, I suggest that the concept of the plasticity of the brain is central to an understanding of the value of dreams and I explore some of the neurophysiological processes that underpin this plasticity.

I then review our understanding of the process of working analytically with dreams in the light of this. I will illustrate with dreams from several patients interleaved with material concerning the dreaming process. Throughout I seek to demonstrate the way in which the total interactive, intersubjective experience in the analytic dyad as analyst and patient work with these dreams enables the development of the emotional scaffolding necessary for the process of 'coming into mind'. I suggest that dreams dreamt as an integral part of an analysis have a vital part to play in the process of transforming the effects of poor early relational experience on mind, not only in the contribution they bring to the analytic dialogue, but particularly in the development of the patient's own internal analyst.

The value of dreams and the dreaming process

Rossi (2004) and Ribeiro (2004) argue the value of dreams and the dreaming process. Just as negative states of emotional arousal can lead to the overproduction of stress proteins and illness, so positive psychological experiences can facilitate gene expression, neurogenesis, problem solving and healing (Rossi 2004: 54). Rossi (2004) cites research that shows that when experimental animals experience novelty, environmental enrichment and physical exercise, zif-268, a learning-related gene, is expressed in their REM (dream) sleep, leading to growth and change in the very structure of the pathways in the mind-brain. I suggest that the plasticity of the brain in response to the experiences of the day is central to an understanding of the value of dreams.

Ribeiro emphasizes the value of dream-dependent insight, citing examples from the world of art and science, adding that 'while the biological mechanisms underlying sleep-dependent insight still remain unknown, the available subjective reports of the phenomenon point to an important role of dreams' (Ribeiro 2004: 12). He concludes that 'the function of dreams is to trim and shape the memories acquired during waking, in a cyclic process of creation, selection and generalization of conjectures about the world' (Ribeiro 2004: 12). Here it seems to me that he is describing part of the task of the internal analyst.

Ribeiro (2004: 1) describes dreams as 'hyper-associative strings of fragmented memories that simulate past events and future expectations'. I would like to present a dream concerned with change, with movement, a dream that is in some ways the epitome of the function of dreams and the dreaming process. It is a dream that looks both backward and forward, not only indicating to the dreamer aspects of the self that she might move on to realize, but also indicating the need to explore the past, the shadow, that which is unconsciously known in order to do so.

Xanthe

The patient, a woman in her late thirties, is married and has children. She is a high achiever, a successful career woman with a first-class degree. She struggles with quite a fierce super-ego; perhaps in compensation she chose extra training in order to be able to work with dysfunctional families. She had come to once a week therapy for a number of years. After much thought, and feeling that the children were now old enough for her to be able to manage it, she began to consider entering a four times a week analysis. She wanted it to be for herself but she knew there was also a serious possibility that she might later seek to train as an analyst. We spoke about what both might entail. After the session she went home and that night dreamt the following dream:

> I was looking for a house. I was on the top of the bus, with a companion, near an open space. It seemed to be the unenclosed area of parkland in the centre of the city that I knew well from childhood. On one side was the buildings of the university. On the far side was my school and below it a rather run-down part of the town. The bus paused at the crossroads, waiting for the green light, I looked down and, right on the corner at the crossroads, I saw the beautiful facade of a double-fronted Georgian house. I felt seriously interested in buying the house. We got off the bus and went to have a look. My companion began to show me around the outside. At the side was a row of stables. There were six boxes each with a horse looking out of it. They would each require care. I went round the back and was not entirely surprised to find that the back of the building was in a state of

disrepair. However I felt it was not beyond repair. I was still seriously interested in purchasing it, in getting the chance to live in it.

Jung reminds us that

> The evolutionary stratification of the psyche is more clearly discernible in the dream than in the conscious mind. In the dream the psyche speaks in images, and gives expression to instincts that derive from the most primitive levels of nature. Therefore, through the assimilation of unconscious contents, the momentary life of consciousness can once more be brought into harmony with the law of nature . . . and the patient can be led back to the natural law of his own being.
>
> (Jung 1954a: para. 351)

In this dream we may note the impressive persona of this patient as reflected in the impressive facade of the building contrasting strongly with what is at first unseen, which is the back of the building in such a state of disrepair with stabled horses representing the need for drive and energy to be cared for. While looking down from the bus reflects the patient's tendency to retreat into defensive objectivity, I was heartened to hear that the dreamer had alighted from the bus and with a companion (whom she later identified to me as 'probably you') had begun to explore the building more closely, thus demonstrating commitment to the kind of journey that Jung proposes.

I asked what my patient had made of the dream. She told the dream again, adding that the price tag had been £6 million! She felt it was expensive but should nevertheless be seriously considered. She said, 'I thought of the six million dollar man, he got destructed, his past was gone'; smiling broadly she added,

> but then he was made anew and he could do anything! Maybe that's what happens in four times a week analysis, that's expensive too, isn't it? Only he was a robotic man and the aim of analysis would not be to become robotic! We [my patient and her husband] talked about the training and how expensive that might be, but I found I was still interested. I am lucky in that we could manage financially. Hmm £6 million!

She continued: 'I don't know about the horses'.

I commented: 'I think we did mention six years of analysis'. She replied:

> Oh yes that's right and then I thought about analysis being to do with feelings, with the passions and thought maybe that's what the horses are about, you know in Plato, I think it's in Phaedrus, about the horses as passions, about driving in the sky.

Later as I remembered how my patient had become more animated I found myself thinking of Jung's description of the horse as 'dynamic and vehicular power: [that] carries one away like a surge of instinct' (Jung 1954: para. 347) and Hillman's comment that 'animals wake up the imagination . . . that animal dreams provoke . . . feelings . . . make us more instinctually alive' (Hillman and McLean 1997: 2) and of the horse in particular: 'we forget how they belong to the airy element as if all horses had wings, flying through the wind, tail streaming, nostrils flared wide' (Hillman and McLean 1997: 47). But I also remembered that for the moment the horses in Xanthe's dream were stabled, but not yet owned, requiring care and attention.

In the next session Xanthe began to talk about the area where the house was. She experienced it as an area where opposites met: on one side her father's world of the university contrasting strongly with the other side of the park with her school and below it a rather seedy part of the city, a shadow area where she was uncertain whether to venture, in fact she knew her parents would not have wished her to explore it.

We went on to explore a little of her fears concerning the nature of analysis, her fear of me as an analyst who might treat her in the way the robotic man was treated, the reminder it carried of her parents' overdetermined way of controlling her future, who she would be, where she might study (at 8 years old she had known which Oxbridge college her parents had in mind for her), what she might become, and how she might fear I would be like that with her if she came to analysis four times a week.

Jacoby (1969) notes that a dream may provide 'imagery, which can often be used with great pertinence with the patient since the imagery stems from her own fantasy world ... the dream also shows her unconscious expectation of [the analyst]' (Jacoby 1969: 141). Fonagy (2000: 92) comments that 'it is now widely recognised that there is a critical transferential aspect to the interpretation of dreams ... dreams are not produced in isolation but are rather dreamt with the analyst in mind'.

As Jung stressed, emotional truth underpins the dreaming process and as dreams are recalled in the consulting-room this may be experienced by the analyst in the countertransference. Through work with dreams within the analytic dyad, new entities are added to pre-existing connections in both brain-minds. I will return to this theme later in the chapter but first I wish to examine some research into the activity of dreaming and the nature of the process.

Jung's attitude shows remarkable compatibility with current understanding of the neuropsychology of the process. Jung understood so clearly that dreams do not lie but communicate the emotional truth as it is: such insight is confirmed by the latest research in neuroscience. In contrast the Freudian concepts of disguise and censorship have come into question.

What then is dreaming?

Dreaming is caused by brain activity during sleep that is both biochemically and regionally different from that of waking states. As early as 1968, Kirsch drew attention to the significance of dream research for the analytic world noting the research of Aserinsky, Kleitman and many others and urged 'the need for a reassessment of our psychological understanding of dreams based on the recent research' (Kirsch 1968: 1462). In 1953 Aserinsky and Kleitman discovered that the brain-mind exhibited periodic self-activation during sleep, these periods of activity, which occurred every 90 to 100 minutes, were accompanied by rapid eye movements and acute accelerations of the heart and respiration rates. When sleepers were wakened and asked to report it was found that REM sleep was characterized by longer, more bizarre and vivid dream accounts than those given on waking from non-rapid eye movement (NREM) sleep. Such studies have been replicated many times over. Solms and Turnbull summarize: '90–95% of awakenings from REM sleep produce dream reports, whereas only 5–10% of awakenings from NREM produce equivalent reports' (Solms and Turnbull 2002: 183).

Studies based on PET scans do indeed reveal the highly selective regional activation pattern of the brain of REM sleep. Major groups of researchers note that in REM sleep the limbic system, especially the amygdala, is activated while the frontal or executive areas of the brain are deactivated. They therefore assign to REM sleep a significant role in the processing of emotion. It comes as no surprise that the regional activation shown in these imaging studies confirms what analysts have long known, namely, that dreams are the mind's vehicle for the processing of emotional states of being, particularly the fear, anger, anxiety or elation that figure prominently in dreams, the passions represented in Xanthe's dream by the six horses to which she would need to give attention.

What is happening now is that these recent imaging studies are confirming just why we do what we do as Jungian analysts, that is concentrate on the mood and affect that underpin the dream, and the relation of this to the dreamer's waking emotional life and ways of relating. Hobson describes dreams as 'the transparent exposure of an individual's cognitive associations to, and means of coping with, anxiety' (Hobson 1999: 170). He urges the therapist to ignore the bizarreness and instead to attend to the undisguised emotional content. Hobson comments that the results from research do not support in any way the Freudian notion of disguise. His concept of the dream process is that it reveals rather than hides the 'emotionally salient concerns' of the dreamer's mind. As Jung commented:

> Dreams do not deceive, they do not lie, they do not distort or disguise, but naively announce what they are and what they mean . . . they are invariably seeking to express something that the ego does not know and does not understand.
>
> (Jung 1946: para. 189)

Hobson (1999) concludes that anxiety, elation and anger are the major shapers of dream plots and adds:

> for the reform-minded psychoanalyst, this should be heard as brain-music of divine inspiration because it suggests that dreaming is a conscious state in which the impact of emotion on cognition is more clearly demonstrated than in waking.
>
> (Hobson 1999: 170)

Braun (1999) notes that REM sleep constitutes in the cortex a unique condition of information processing functionally isolated from input from the external world or output to it. The dream is therefore in a unique way the expression of the internal, the intra-psychic world of the dreamer (Braun 1999). Dream logic ignores logical aspects of conscious thought in a way that often takes dreamers by surprise if they waken and are able to recall their dream. Reiser (1999) emphasizes the subjective nature of dreaming which he characterizes as 'the subjective experience in dream con-sciousness of vital memory and cognitive operations made possible by the special psychophysiological conditions that obtain in mind/ brain-body during REM and comparably activated brain states during sleep' (Reiser 1999: 205). Again the dream may be under-stood as stimulating the development of the internal analyst.

Despite the amnesia associated with dreaming, it has become clear that dreaming has a vital role to play in the affective organisa-tion of memory. Reiser draws our attention to 'the principle of affective organisation of memory' (Reiser 1999: 203). He explains:

> Each of us carries within the mind-brain an enduring network of stored memories encoded by images ... perceived during significant emotional life experiences. Such images and the memories they encode are associationally linked by a shared potential to evoke identical or highly similar complexes of emo-tion. Such networks are organised around a core of perceptual images or part images that encode memories of early events.
>
> (Reiser 1999: 203)

The corticolimbic circuits make sorting decisions on a pattern-matching basis, enabling learning by cumulative experience. The brain regions responsible for this activity have been shown to be highly activated in REM sleep. The most elegant exposition of the relation of Jung's theory of archetypes and this kind of early encoding is to be found in Jean Knox's (2003) book *Archetype, Attachment, Analysis: Jungian psychology and the emergent mind.*

It now no longer surprises me, as it would once have done, to discover Panksepp, a neuroscientist, arguing that the underlying emotional circuits of the brain '*initiate, synchronise* and *energise* sets of coherent physiological, behavioural and psychological changes that are primal instinctive solutions to various archetypal life-challenging situations' (Panksepp 1998: 123, italics in original). He argues that REM sleep permits information processing whereby transient memory stores become integrated into subconscious behavioural habits, adding, 'Perhaps the dream theories of Freud and Jung, which suggested dreams reflect unconscious and symbolic emotional forces affecting an individual may still hold some basic truths' (Panksepp 1998: 129). He concludes that REM sleep may help

> to solidify the many unconscious habits that are the very foundation of our personality. In the final accounting dreams may construct the powerful subconscious or preconscious affective psychological patterns that make us . . . the people that we are. They may help construct the many emotional myths and beliefs around which our lives revolve.
>
> (Panksepp 1998: 142)

Here it would seem that Panksepp attributes an emergent archetypal aspect to the function of REM sleep.

Brain imaging studies reveal that

> vivid visual dreams light up the visual cortex; nightmares trigger activity in the amygdala and the hippocampus flares up from time to time to relay recent events. The areas which seem to be most commonly active are the pathways carrying alerting signals from the brainstem and the auditory cortex; supplementary motor areas and visual association areas – all of which produce the 'virtual reality effect of dreaming'.
>
> (Carter 2000: 318)

The function of certain zones is diametrically reversed during dream sleep, for example activity is decreased in the dorsolateral prefrontal cortex, the area of waking thought and reality testing and inhibition rather than excitation is actively promoted in the areas of the brain concerned with motor activity (Carter 2000; Panksepp 1998).

What light is then shed on the purpose of dreams?

Hobson and Pace-Schott (1999), as a result of large-scale studies, conclude that dreaming consciousness contrasts with waking consciousness in that the brain is activated in a bottom-up manner rather than the top-down mode of waking thought. In dreaming ascending activity begins in the brain stem, progresses through the limbic system, reaching the medial frontal cortex (which deals with arousal and attention). They note that the executive portions of the frontal cortex (i.e. the dorsolateral cortex and the orbito prefrontal cortex) are deactivated. They conclude: 'dreaming cognition is bizarre because of the loss of the organising capacity of the brain, not because of an elaborate disguise mechanism that rids an internal stimulus of an unacceptable meaning' (Hobson and Pace-Schott 1999: 211).

REM sleep is a unique condition of internal information processing without reference to input from the outside world. The analyst may truly understand the dream as a reflection of the patient's internal world, as indeed Xanthe's dream of the Georgian house reflected her self-experience.

Studies by Hobson have led to greater understanding of the specific effects in relation to REM sleep of certain neuromodulators. Key chemicals in the brain are thought to influence the dreaming process, and the debate concerning clarity or censorship as the purpose of the dream rages around their relative roles. Neurotransmitters are chemicals that transmit messages from brain cell to brain cell, that is from neuron to neuron, and some neurotransmitters are also neuromodulators that modify effects in the brain. Of particular significance for the understanding of the dreaming brain-mind are *dopamine* involved in curiosity-interest-expectancy responses and the dreaming process, *norepinephrine* involved in the brain's emergency response to trauma, and *serotonin* which regulates mood and emotion.

Hobson (1999) emphasizes that in waking states the noradrenergic and serotinergic systems are on and the cholinergic system is dampened, and that in REM sleep just the opposite pertains, that is the noradrenergic and serotinergic systems are dampened and the cholinergic system is dominant. Hobson notes that norepinephrine and serotonin drop almost to zero in REM sleep whereas acetylcholine release is enhanced because the inhibitory constraint of acetylcholine exercised by norepinephrine and serotonin during periods of wakefulness is diminished. Reduced serotonin in REM sleep has been demonstrated in the amygdala, hippocampus, orbitofrontal cortex and the cingulate cortex. This implies that the 'human limbic system is turned on but demodulated during dreaming' (Hobson 1999: 164).

Hobson's conclusions, while congruent with Jung's view of

dreaming, are at odds with the classical Freudian concepts of disguise and censorship. Solms marshals a defence for the classical Freudian view of the dream as a disguised and denied wish (Solms 1999; Solms and Turnbull 2002: 211–16). Solms stresses the importance of the activation of the dopamine circuit in the brain at the time of dreaming and argues that it is this, rather than the dominance of the cholinergic system, that gives rise to all peculiar states of dream-like experience, including actual dreaming. He suggests that this activates the system that Panksepp has described as the seeking circuit that is characterized by curiosity and eagerness causing the sleeping ego to protest against the seeming wish fulfilment of the dream state. One may, however, question the capacity of the ego to achieve this in view of the deactivation of much of what Solms would be the first to acknowledge as the executive brain. I would add that Solms' thesis has arisen from observation of the effects of damage to particular areas of the brain in a very small sample group of patients.

Nevertheless this aspect of Solms' work is of particular interest for our understanding of the dreaming mind-brain as it demonstrates the six areas of the brain that are crucially involved in the dreaming process. Kaplan-Solms and Solms' (2000) method of study is underpinned by that developed by the Russian neurologist Luria, who argued that lesions in different parts of the brain disturb function in different ways. Luria (1987) concluded that by careful observation of patients with particular lesions the component parts of each functional system might be identified and localized in different tissues of the brain. This method known as 'dynamic localization', based on intensive study of patients with cerebral lesions, forms the basic research tool for Kaplan-Solms and Solms' (2000) work. They see it as a vital bridge between neuropsychology and psychoanalysis as it makes possible the identification of the neurological organization of any mental faculty, without contradicting the tenets of psychoanalysis. By using this method of research they are able to show the effect on the dreaming process of local damage in six specific areas of the brain.

Kaplan-Solms and Solms (2000) delineate the three areas, damage to any one of which will lead to loss of the capacity to dream. They emphasize with each area that while it affects a particular ability, that particular area is only one of several regions in the brain whose concerted action is responsible for that particular ability. Left parietal lobe lesions will affect the ability for abstraction, concept formation and symbolization and will lead to loss of dreaming. Right parietal damage gives rise to defects in visual-spatial working memory and thus to loss of dreaming. Damage to the ventromesial white matter of the front lobes results in loss of spontaneous motivation and with it the capacity to dream one's dream, indicating that with Freud (and also Jung), dreaming must be understood as a meaningful event. More subtle disturbances of dreaming are also noted in that ventromesial occipito-temporal damage gives rise to dreams devoid of imagery, frontal limbic damage results in loss of the ability to distinguish between dreams and reality and temporal lobe seizure equivalents give rise to stereo-typed nightmare dreams which also appear in the form of waking seizures and aurae and disappear in response to appropriate medi-cation or surgery. Using the method of dynamic localization as a conceptual bridge between neuropsychology and psychoanalysis, they are thus able to demonstrate that dreaming is a dynamic pro-cess unfolding over a functional system that has six component parts (Kaplan-Solms and Solms 2000).

Braun (1999), in reviewing the wider debate in the light of his own and other research findings, argues that neither the cholin-ergic nor the dopaminergic hypothesis will prove to be the sole explanation of the dreaming process (Braun 1999: 196–200). He emphasizes the common ground among the protagonists and stresses that 'the activation of the limbic system, in the absence of top-down control by the frontal cortex, provides a context in which salient memories and emotions are manifest' (Braun 1999: 198). He warns against an 'either' 'or' approach to understanding the chemical aspects of the dreaming process, and also suggests that neither theory will prove to be sufficient explanation concerning the dreaming process. Rather he argues that the pattern of activity may actually be driven 'by differential patterns of information transfer between cortex and thalamus, perhaps coordinated by the reticular nucleus' or, he continues, 'the pattern may be "set" within cortical networks themselves' (Braun 1999: 198).

One might ask what common ground is there among the researchers. What has become increasingly clear is that dreams pro-cess states of emotion, that dreams have meaning and that REM sleep appears to play an important role in the organization of mem-ory. I would like to emphasize that, with Braun (1999), we should assume that the meaning of the dream is mapped on its surface, not disguised and in need of decoding. Indeed Braun himself comments that he is rather inclined to agree with Jung, who said, 'I am doubtful whether we can assume a dream is something other than it appears to be' (Jung 1938: para. 41). I conclude that, as clinicians, we should take note of Jung's recommendation that 'we should not pare down the meaning of the dream to fit some narrow doctrine' (Jung 1954: para. 318) but rather we should appreciate that

> the 'manifest' dream picture is the dream itself and contains the whole meaning of the dream ... What Freud calls the 'dream-façade' is the dream's obscurity, and this is really only a projection of our own lack of understanding ... We say that the dream has a false front only because we fail to see into it.
>
> (Jung 1954: para. 319)

A contemporary Jungian approach to dream analysis

Clinical illustration of the compatibility of Hobson (1999), Braun (1999) and Reiser's (1999) view of dreaming with a contemporary Jungian approach to dream analysis may be seen in the following dream material. It demonstrates the way that the total interactive experience within the analytic dyad over time and reflected in work with dream series rather than individual dreams (Jung 1954: para. 322), enables the development of the emotional scaffolding necessary for the emergence of reflective function, for 'coming into mind'. The patients that follow both experienced a mother who was unable to allow her baby to attach in a healthy way that would call forth the baby's capacity to engage, to separate and to develop a healthy capacity to self-regulate. Both had fathers who were absent much of the time and who were unable to offer emotional support to the mother–baby dyad. These early experiences dictated the nature of their internal objects, the contents of their inner world. Thus it is the inner world, experienced in the transference, that the analyst must address in dream work rather than be tempted to examine dreams of trauma patients merely in a reductive or reconstructive manner.

Susan

I would like to return to Susan, who I introduced in Chapter 4, in order to look at some of her dreams. As we have already seen, Susan experienced a prolonged separation from her mother from the age of 6 weeks to 18 months and then at 18 months experienced the almost total loss of the single aunt who came and stayed in their home and who had acted as the primary caretaker during that time. At about 3 years old, she was again separated from her mother; this time she was sent to stay with cousins some distance away. She experienced abuse by her uncle while with this family. It is not clear how long this stay was. She never told her much-loved aunt or her mother: her uncle had told her that if she told someone that person would die. She seems to have put the experience almost entirely out of mind. She came into analysis in her thirties because of increasing feelings of intense anxiety. Unknown to her conscious mind, her daughter was approaching the age Susan had been when she was sexually abused. The first six months of the analysis was a time of increasingly regressive experiences in the consulting-room bringing increasing awareness of a huge amount of 'unknown' early distress. As the work became securely established, Susan's experiences that had been put entirely out of mind began to emerge in many vivid dreams that elaborated a repetitive dream that Susan had experienced since childhood. With hindsight it became apparent that the dreams addressed more and more clearly split-off, unconscious contents of the psyche.

Dream 1

She was trying to escape from a young, dark-haired man who was in pursuit of her. She had a child with her. There were long corridors, perhaps a hospital environment, perhaps a school. She was surrounded by lots of people whose faces were very alive but who behaved as spectators, neither helping nor harming.

Susan contrasted this version of the dream with her childhood repetitive nightmare. This dream was in colour and peopled in contrast to the childhood nightmare, in which she fled alone down dark subterranean passages, or across dark, lonely landscapes. In the childhood version she was the child running away from an unseen threat. In her adult dream she tried to help the child as they both fled from the young, dark-haired man. Years later she was to find a photograph of her uncle from that time and brought it to analysis. It showed not the overweight, elderly bald man that she thought of as her uncle, but the young dark-haired man of her dream.

The walled-off, dissociated nature of this psychic splinter, or traumatic complex, was reflected in another from the prolific dream series originating from this period of the analysis.

Dream 2

She was chased by a man who somehow seemed more substantial. She ran over walkways with stagnant water either side. There was a danger she would fall in, a danger that she would be caught. The walkway was over a lake. It led to a walled-off stretch of stagnant water. As she found herself there she woke in terror.

As the analysis progressed there was a subtle shift of direction, a sense of something walled-off which she was approaching but as yet had not faced, a sense of being taken ineluctably to a known but, as yet unthought, destination. Dreams which occurred several months later, at the point where it had become possible to increase Susan's sessions to three times a week, reflected this clearly.

Dream 3

She went into the Underground. There were new silver trains. She boarded an old maroon train that had been standing in a siding for a long while. The train set off towards her destination, it had no lights. There were black figures of men further up the train, one or another would suddenly lean out of the train at an angle, then lean back again. She was terrified it would crash. Her fear woke her.

She fell asleep again almost immediately and dreamt again.

Dream 4

Men on horseback came towards her from all directions. There was a gun. She was frightened of the gun. It was possessed by different men. She was frightened it would be used on her.

Again she woke in terror.

Susan was no longer running away from the destructive, aggressive aspects of her inner world but rather was moving towards, or was surrounded by, material emerging from the unconscious in response to the deepening transference. This change of direction, towards greater conscious knowing of the walled-off, unknowable, experience that had been put entirely out of mind continued to emerge in many vivid dreams. This powerful healing process felt to her as if it arose from deep within her; analysis of it made possible the retrieval of feeling and memory, and released major amounts of energy for living that had previously been devoted to keeping the unthinkable out of mind.

What then do I understand as dream analysis?

What is it that is actually being explored when analyst and analysand work together on such dreams? Ribeiro (2004) argues that the repetitive dreams of the trauma patient eliminate once and for all any suggestion that dreams are the result of random cortical activation. Rather he stresses that 'recursive nightmares are an important symptom of post-traumatic stress disorder, which is characterised by disturbed, hyper-aroused REM-sleep' (Ribeiro 2004: 4). Trauma has been shown to result in impaired development of the corpus callosum (Teicher 2000); such a functional disconnection leads to disavowal. Pally (2000: 132) comments that such 'patients can speak about emotional events but deny their emotional significance'. Dream work over time may actually help to reverse such effects, encouraging inter- and intra-hemispheric connectivity.

Dreaming is essentially a cortical activity in that it is the cortex with its billions of connecting neurons that allows us to experience the richness of thoughts and imagery that emerge from the dreaming process. In working with dreams in general, not just those dreams arising from trauma, the individual develops the creative capacity to make conceptual and affective links across different realms of knowing; material may begin to move from unconscious implicit memory towards the explicit realm of knowledge and memory.

Jung describes a similar process in relation to dream analysis when he argues the need for assimilation rather than free association in the analyst's approach to the patient's dreams. He defines assimilation as a 'mutual penetration of conscious and unconscious' (Jung 1954: para. 327). He emphasizes that threat from the unconscious diminishes as soon as the patient begins to assimilate contents that were previously unconscious (Jung 1954: para. 329). Jung concludes: 'That is why every dream is an organ of information and control, and why dreams are our most effective aid in building up the personality' (Jung 1954: para. 332). Dream work is therefore an essentially integrative process in the brain.

But how does this come about? Dreams may be thought of as extended symbolic metaphors. Jung argues that dream symbols should not be understood as 'signs or symptoms' but as 'true symbols, i.e., as expressions of a content not yet consciously recognized or conceptually formulated' (Jung 1954: para. 339). I find the work of Levin (1997) and Modell (1997) (both cited in Pally 2000) particularly significant in regard to this, emphasizing as it does that metaphor lights up multiple centres in the brain enabling increased connectivity in the brain. Indeed Solms suggests that consciousness itself may be understood as the connectivity established in the individual brain-mind (Solms in debate with Greenfield 2002).

Dream metaphor reflects the particular preoccupations of the dreamer and the underlying complexes that drive these preoccupations. Hartmann stresses that 'as we move along our continuum from focused waking thought – to dreaming, our mental processes become increasingly metaphoric' (Hartmann 2000: 69–70). He argues that a dream provides 'the explanatory metaphor for the dominant emotion or concern of the dreamer' (Hartmann 2000: 69–70). As such, dreams reflect particular patterns of neural connectedness in the dreamer's brain. Much use of metaphor is synaesthetic, reflecting the underlying neural nets in the brain-mind. Such emergent metaphor stimulates the possibility of an encounter with the unconscious in a powerful way for metaphor has been found to light up more centres in the brain than any other form of human communication. Dream metaphor may be experienced synaesthetically as the normal functions of logical thought and processing vanish in the face of vivid dream experiences. Hartmann (2000) suggests that this is because the neural nets that are activated in the dreaming process are looser than the more tightly woven nets that deal with the linguistic or mathematical functioning of the awake and focused mind. The dreaming mind-brain's use of emergent metaphor allows the possibility of an encounter between conscious and unconscious, such as Jung envisaged; such an encounter with the symbolic facilitates the individuation process. Jung likened the dream to a theatre in which 'the dreamer is himself the scene, the player, the prompter, the producer, the author, the public and the critic' (Jung 1960: para. 509).

Cambray and Carter (2004: 130) describe dream analysis as a 'co-constructed process evolving within in an on-going, containing relationship'. In the context of work concerning early relational trauma it is this containing relationship that makes it possible to dream the undreamable as a prelude to becoming able to think the unthinkable, and as a prelude to recreating experience not in terms of the historical past but in terms of the relational present. Covington (1995) urges the necessity for a distinction to be made 'between historical reconstruction within the transference and the establishment of history within the analytic frame itself . . . [where] the present takes centre stage while at the same time remaining influenced by the past' (Covington 1995: 410). She argues that this distinction holds within it the possibility of 'a transference in which the future self of the patient emerges' (Covington 1995: 410). Her arguments, although addressed to work with narrative in the consulting-room, are equally applicable to the material that emerges from the dreaming process. Past is revisited at the level of the implicit and moves towards the explicit, changing deeply founded ways of being and behaving, leading to change in the nature of attachment. Cambray and Carter (2004), understanding the dream as a communication of a psychic state at a particular moment, emphasize that 'critical for therapeutic value is that the dreamer discovers/recovers in the analytic process the affective experience residing in the dream' (Cambray and Carter 2004: 131). The dream will in a sense be experienced together as implicit speaks to implicit in the analytic dyad. Out of this shared experience well-timed verbal interpretations may develop enabling implicit to become explicit. Beebe (2005) urges care in the way in which we interpret, and illustrates his point by identifying three different kinds of nightmares each requiring a different sort of response from the analyst. Both aspects of the analytic process, that is the implicit relational and the explicit interpretational, are fostered by work with dreams and form an intrinsic part of the process of coming into mind.

Cambray and Carter (2004: 121) urge that 'the approach used to enter and engage symbolic reality must . . . seek to stay near the creative edge'. Emergent metaphor such as is encountered in the dreaming process stimulates the possibility of an encounter with the unconscious expressed in a powerful way through vivid images. For some patients dream images may at first be

> thought of as a transitional experience that allows the potential linking of self-states that are . . . disconnected, permitting the voices of other self-states to be heard and to find access to the dynamic structure the patient defines as me.
>
> (Bromberg 2000: 694)

For some this may be most easily conveyed through a visual image, and then with difficulty in the safety of the consulting-room that image may come to be formulated in words and felt.

Holly

This patient, a woman in her mid-forties, was one of several professional artists I have seen over the years. Holly experienced extremely potent visual dream images; at one point the easiest way for her to convey these was through making images. Plates 1–3 show some of these images. At the time these were made, our work was dominated by Holly's experience of me as the hostile, persecuting, destructive mother analyst: I carried the projection of her internalized destructive and persecuting mother. It seems that the internal mother was very much in the image of her own mother. Her mother in her turn had received inadequate parenting that had meant there was no good enough mother for her to internalize, which would have enabled her to parent Holly in a more nurturing way. In the sessions as we worked together, in a moment it seemed, she would suddenly change, her face would for a moment show fear, and then would become hard as she closed off completely from me. Almost a whole session would pass, as she would struggle with her experience of me as the bad mother. Wordlessness was the most striking feature of her state of being at these times as she became dominated by right brain functioning, by deeply held ways of being and behaving arising out of the traumatic quality of her earliest relational experience, lodged deep in implicit (right brain) memory. A turning point came when Holly went home and painted a picture of a dream of a fearsome black cat mauling a baby cat (see Plate 1). It filled her with fear, but she was able to bring it to the session and it enabled her to engage the left hemisphere of the brain as she thought about material emerging from the right. Haltingly she was able to discuss her uncertainty about whether I was the bad black cat mother attacking her, or whether she was the bad black cat tearing me to shreds. Hillman reminds us that 'the dream animal shows us that the imagination has jaws and paws, that it can wake us in the night with panic and terror or move us to tears' (Hillman 1997: 24). So through the image we became able to talk about how aggression becomes internalized, how experience both of being abused and being the abuser inhabited her internal world. Towards the end of the session we noticed a little cream cat, which we felt symbolized the child carrying the hope. This little cat is uncannily like my much-loved little female cat that the patient has never seen or known about consciously. She then brought a second painting which she felt came from a very different place in her. It combined elements of the garden outside the consulting-room with good elements of her own garden (see Plate 2). The hard edge of the moor above my consulting-room, which had terrified her on her first visit, had become merged with the garden fence. The edge had become a happy place where people walked freely, as indeed it is in reality.

Patients find it difficult to overcome fear and may cling to an experience with the analyst that feels good and containing. Fear and rage mingle together and often may only be experienced in projection, and as such mean that the analyst may suddenly be experienced as a frighteningly sadistic part object at any time. Susan, mentioned earlier (p. 143), brought further dreams that illustrated this and these provided opportunities to work with both idealized and persecutory aspects of the transference.

Susan

Dream 5

She dreamt of a beautiful container with fresh, clear water bubbling up in it. As she lent forward to take a drink she could see a hand reaching up towards her under the water. She stretched out her hand to touch the fingers. Suddenly it turned into a fierce piranha fish which began to eat her fingers. She took her hand out of the container but four fingers were gone.

Two further dreams illustrate the same sort of struggle.

Dream 6 'Red Riding Hood'

I went to visit my analyst, or my much-loved grandmother. I looked into her face only to find it had become that of a bear or a wolf. I woke terrified.

Dream 7 'The penis analyst'

The analyst and I went into a theatre together. Just as we were finding our way to our seats I gave a pretend growl. She immediately changed into a hugely tall, narrow, ribbed, pinky, fawny, grey figure. I woke myself with my scream of fear.

Quinodoz's work on paradoxical dreams is relevant here. He suggests that some dreams that include an 'anxiety-inducing primitive content that frightens the dreamer' (Quinodoz 2002: 3) may actually indicate the fulfilment of a stage of psychic integration, albeit that the content focuses on the regressive internal situation that has just been overcome. Quinodoz speculates that such dreams indicate a coming-together of split-off parts returning to the dreamer's self (Quinodoz 2002: 47).

For Susan, by the close of her analysis the transference experience had changed considerably and Susan's dreams reflected this new perspective, which reflected the pivotal shift that had taken place in her internal world.

Dream 8 (Susan called this dream 'The new internal couple')

Susan was on a journey with a couple who treated her as if she were their daughter. They were sharing a cabin and Susan was in a single bed. Just across the room, the mother was also in bed. She was peaceful and smiled at Susan. She was a dark-haired Italian-looking woman with a creamy skin. She reminded Susan of both her analyst and a mother. The father came into the room and she sensed his kindness. She was suddenly aware she was very small as he spoke to her and lifted her up in a gentle way, noticing her stiffness and enabling her to relax. As he did so she was aware that her aunt, who had also come into the room behind him, was slipping quietly out of the door. As her aunt left, Susan awoke.

As Susan reflected in the session on what she had dreamt so near the end of her analysis, she was able to realize that now there was an image of a new parental couple within she no longer needed analysis in the special way she had. In childhood her aunt had been the only one to keep alive the knowledge of Susan's true self in her internal world, now the work had enabled Susan's true self to emerge and to flourish.

Stewart (1992) describes beautifully the relation of inner and outer, of transference experience and dream image:

> It is from the development of external personal relationships in the transference, where experiences of space, mobility and separateness arise, that internalisation of these processes and experiences occur to give rise to experiences of internal space, mobility and separateness as manifested in these dream experiences.
>
> (Stewart 1992: 39)

Conclusion

I hope that the dreams that I have invited you to consider as we have moved through the chapter have provided clinical illustration of the compatibility of a neuroscientific view of dreaming with a contemporary Jungian approach to dream analysis. The dreams speak for themselves, revealing the emotionally salient concerns of the dreamers, weaving past and present, transference and reality together in a way that demonstrates the healthy attempt of the mind to pattern match and in this way to come to terms with difficult emotional experience from the past. The dreams became dreamable only within the emotionally supportive context of the analytic relationship.

Sherwood (2005) argues the need for a sophisticated approach to dreaming, noting that Jungians are in 'a unique position to speak about the nature of dreams, because [they] have been working with dreams and exploring their reality for quite a while now'. She suggests the formation of a working group 'to explore the interface between our literature on dreaming and the neuroimaging research and to open up a dialogue with dream researchers' (Sherwood 2005). As dream research continues, with I predict, Gamwell, that the twenty-first century will have available 'a new concept of dreamwork that fully integrates neurology with the subjective experience of self [and that it will carry] the serious stamp of science' (Gamwell 2000: 55) that both Freud and Jung so desired.

Chapter 9

The emergent self

> The birth of the personality in oneself has a therapeutic value. It is as if a river that had run to waste in sluggish side-streams and marshes suddenly found its way back to its proper bed, or as if a stone lying on a germinating seed were lifted away so that the shoot could begin its natural growth. The inner voice is the voice of a fuller life, of a wider, more comprehensive consciousness.
>
> (Jung 1954c: para. 317–18)

The last area I have chosen to look at is the self. I wish to explore the relevance of insights from neuroscience that lead to my understanding of the emergence of self as a process that is contingent on relationship to another, an understanding of the self as relational. I understand the very basis of self to be associative, arising out of a hard-wired disposition to relate to another, evident at birth and in the earliest days of life. Because the self emerges from experiences of relating, a healthy sense of self is contingent upon good experience with the primary care-giver. Very poor early experience leads not so much to repression, although in milder circumstances that may occur, but rather to dissociated self-states that may vary in the degree of severity, with the far end of the spectrum being the manifestations of multiplicity found in dissociative identity disorder. Thus my emphasis is not on experience that arises endogenously from the action of drives as in classical Freudian theory but rather exogenously from empathic relating by the primary care-giver, initially experienced bodily and which gives rise to increasing connectivity in the brain. Thus the view of self-consciousness is one of increasing connectivity in good enough circumstances, or disconnectedness where there has been an experience that is inadequate.

This accords with Jung's thought throughout his life and with some of Freud's earlier writings but contrasts with his later view of consciousness and unconsciousness as a hierarchical system, in which repression enables the unacceptable to sink out of sight.

The primary associative self

From conception the baby to be depends on another for the ability to develop into a being who will live in relation to others. At birth babies will, if allowed the opportunity, crawl up their mother's tummy themselves to find the nipple; in the process they may look long into the mother's face (Johnson and Johnson 2000). Earlier in the book (Chapter 3) I have described the importance of the mother's face for 2-month-old Jacques. Woodhead (2004) (see Chapter 3) describes the process of 'naming' the baby together as part of her work of helping a traumatized mother to really meet her daughter as a 'psychological self', noting that as this baby looked into her mother's face she was more 'likely to see her mother's preoccupied suffering rather than her [Nadia's] self' (Woodhead 2004: 148–9). Not without reason did Schore describe the mother's face as 'the most potent visual stimulus in the baby's world' (Schore 2002: 18).

From Jung's concept of the self, Fordham (1969) postulated the existence of a primary self, present at birth, which develops by means of a process of deintegration and reintegration as the infant engages and interacts with the outside world. Astor points out that while Fordham's model emphasizes the infant as a separate person it also gives weight to the need for an adequate fit between infant and mother for each sequence of deintegration and reintegration to take place. Astor comments: 'Important in this process was the mother's capacity to receive and make sense of the baby's communication in such a way that the baby took in from its mother's attention . . . that it . . . could be understood' (Astor 1998: 12). In this connection, Tzourio-Mazoyer et al.'s (2002) research has indicated the importance of the mother's face for the development of later social relating, noting that in the early smiling exchanges with mother, and the proto-conversation that accompanies them, babies recruit the area in the left hemisphere that will later become the seat of language.

It is in the area of an understanding of the concept of the self in depth psychology, that a Jungian perspective is perhaps most relevant to the empirical studies in neuroscience that have developed since the beginning of the 1990s, although one must always ask what exactly the writer is meaning by the word 'self'. Jung's notion of the self as a totality, and Fordham's notion of the infant as 'a psychosomatic unity or self' which will contribute by deintegration to all psychic structures as they differentiate in growth are particularly congruent with the work of Damasio (1999), Panksepp (1998) and LeDoux (2002). The notion of the awareness of self as a conscious being with a mind capable of intentionality, desire, belief and emotion is less compatible with the neuroscientists' concept of core self, but is rather in keeping with their view of a sense of self which arises gradually as experience of relating to another builds connectivity into the developing brain. Damasio, for example, suggested a 'preconscious biological precedent', entirely outside of consciousness, that he termed the 'protoself' (Damasio 1999: 153). By this he meant an essentially unconscious bodily based foundation to the self, from which the core self, which we each sense within, may develop. Cambray (2005) observes that both Jung and Damasio reached back into the seventeenth century to ground their thinking about mind-body relations (Jung explored the writings of Leibniz in a similar way to Damasio's more recent quest for insight based on the writings of Descartes and Spinoza). Cambray comments: 'in this view the mind can neither be reduced to brain activity in itself, nor is it a wholly independent agency, the mental world emerges from, or supervenes on the somatic' (Cambray 2005: 197). Thus, as Peter Fonagy reminded us, at the conference held to celebrate the fiftieth anniversary of the Anna Freud Centre, 'the mind is wrongly seen as a mere product of brain function, it is also its determinant . . . the mind must be studied in order to understand the brain' (Fonagy 2002).

Neuroscientists stress the importance of zones of convergence that receive and integrate inputs from many different brain areas. Solms and Turnbull note the particular areas of the upper brain stem that receive input from all the sensory modalities and that produce a 'virtual map' of the musculoskeletal body. They are adjacent to the area where the mapping of inner visceral states takes place. They suggest that these two maps together, mapping 'the inner' and 'the outer', generate a rudimentary representation of the whole person, the inner and outer virtual bodies combined (Solms and Turnbull 2002: 110). It is this region that also leads Panksepp (1998) to posit a coherent foundational process, that he terms the 'self-representation [or] primordial self-schema [that] provides input into many sensory analysers and . . . is strongly influenced by the primal emotional circuits' (Panksepp 1998: 309). He chooses to call this the SELF, by which he means 'a Simple Ego-type Life Form deep within the brain' (Panksepp 1998: 309). He suggests that the SELF first arises during early development from a coherently organized motor process in the subcortical midbrain, even though it comes to be represented in widely distributed ways through the higher regions of the brain as a function of neural and psychological maturation. He continues: 'basic affective states, which initially arise from the changing neurodynamics of a SELF-representation mechanism, may provide an essential psychic scaffolding for all other forms of consciousness' (Panksepp 1998: 309). Thus just as an interactionist developmental view is appropriate for our understanding of archetypal theory, so it is for a full appreciation of the Jungian archetypal view of the self.

In fact, despite Panksepp's choice of Freudian terminology, his understanding of SELF appears to be much closer to that of Jung, who argued that 'The self is not only the centre but also the whole circumference which embraces both conscious and unconscious; it is the centre of this totality, just as the ego is the centre of consciousness' (Jung 1953a: para. 44). He further explains that

> The self is a quantity that is superordinate to the conscious ego. It embraces not only the conscious but also the unconscious psyche, and is therefore, so to speak, a personality which we *also* are . . . There is little hope of our ever being able to reach even approximate consciousness of the self, since however much we may make conscious there will always exist an indeterminate and indeterminable amount of unconscious material which belongs to the totality of the self.
>
> (Jung 1953b: para. 274, italics in original)

The self, manifest in many self-states

LeDoux (2002), in his book *Synaptic Self*, writes: 'the self is the totality of what an organism is physically, biologically, psychologically, socially and culturally' (LeDoux 2002: 31) and in so doing comes close to the Jungian view of the self as a totality. He continues: 'that all aspects of the self are not usually manifest simultaneously and that different aspects can even be contradictory may seem to present a hopelessly complex problem' (LeDoux 2002: 31). He adds:

> different components of the self reflect the operation of different brain systems . . . while explicit memory is mediated by a single system, there are a variety of brain systems that store information implicitly, allowing for many aspects of the self to coexist.
>
> (LeDoux 2002: 31)

Information processing (including interpretations) is highly biased towards the left hemisphere, towards the explicit, declarative, hippocampal field. For our understanding of self-states in patients who have experienced early relational trauma the key will be stored in the implicit, emotional, amygdaloidal memory of the right hemisphere, known only through ways of being, feeling and behaving. Siegel proposes that

> *basic states of mind are clustered into specialised selves, which are enduring states of mind that have a repeating pattern of activity across time* . . . which exist over time with a sense of continuity that creates the experience of mind.
>
> (Siegel 1999: 231, italics in original)

However, Siegel concludes that the successful resolution of the difficulties experienced by those with self-states that are disconnected from one another may not be so much a sense of continuity but 'how the mind integrates a sense of coherence . . . across self-states through time' (Siegel 1999: 231).

Who am I?

But which self is it that we experience at a given moment, and what is the effect of traumatic experience on the development of the self?

I would like to follow Redfearn's example and turn for a moment to the exploration of identity as portrayed by A.A. Milne in the children's classic *Winnie-the-Pooh* (Redfearn 1985). In his seminal book, *My Self, My Many Selves*, Redfearn reminds us that when a rather hungry Winnie-the-Pooh finds himself at the hole of his good friend Rabbit, he goes to call on him, knowing that Rabbit can usually be relied upon for a little honey, and is likely to be willing to listen to the new tune that Winnie-the-Pooh has made up (Milne 1958: 35–6).

When Winnie-the-Pooh first asks if anyone is at home Rabbit, out of nervousness and uncertainty, responds by pretending that he is not there; indeed he claims that Rabbit has gone on a visit to his good friend, Winnie-the-Pooh. All ends well when Pooh Bear manages to convince his friend of his identity and they are reunited (for the complete text, see http://www.poohfriends.com/winniethepooh/thingstoread/chapter2.htm).

Redfearn concludes that

> the establishment of personal identity is a matter of negotiation. The particular identities established are a function of the purpose in hand . . . without our being aware of it, the feeling of 'I' may be taken over first by a hungry Pooh within us, then by a fearful Rabbit and so on. There is a seemingly endless parade of sub-personalities within our total personality, all ready to take the stage and play their allotted roles.
>
> (Redfearn 1985: xi–xii)

Redfearn discusses the internal world of one patient in terms of sub-personalities and observes that the 'figures are "archetypal" in that they occur in many myths, fairy-tales, religious symbols, etc., yet they were very personal and very much part of her peculiar personal history and real life traumata' (Redfearn 1985: 119).

Searles expressed the view that

> The more healthy a person is, the more consciously does he live in the knowledge that there are myriad 'persons' – internal objects each bearing some sense of identity value – within him. He recognises this state of his internal world to be what it is – not threatened insanity, but the strength resident in the human condition.
>
> (Searles 1986: 80, cited in Everest 1999: 460)

Jung understood the more radically split-off or dissociated aspects of personality as 'autonomous splinter psyches' or traumatic complexes which became split off because of traumatic experience (Jung 1934a: para. 203). Jung comments: 'A traumatic complex brings about the dissociation of the psyche. The complex is not under the control of the will and for this reason it possesses the quality of psychic autonomy' (Jung 1928: para. 266). Jung's understanding of these vertical splits, arising out of his work with Charcot and Janet, is much more in keeping with the understanding of those who adopt a relational perspective today than that derived from the later Freud, who renounced the early understanding he too shared with Janet and Charcot in favour of a structural organization that was split horizontally rather than vertically. J.M. Davies (1996) observes that

> the classical unconscious is . . . a repression-based model . . . organised around a developmental layering . . . denoting the history of *endogenously organised*, phase-specific, object-related drives and drive derivatives . . . rather than by *the actual qualities and textures of self-object interactions.*
>
> (Davies 1996: 561, italics in original)

Stolorow reminds us that:

> The problem with classical theory was not its focus on the intrapsychic but its failure to recognise that the intrapsychic world, as it forms within a hierarchy of living, dynamic systems, is exquisitely context-sensitive and context-dependent.
>
> (Stolorow 1997: 866)

Davies (1996) introduces her elegant and discerning article with a description from Masud Khan (1971) of a first session with a patient. He comments:

> She had told her story in a dignified and reticent manner . . . As I looked at her and listened to her I had the same impression as one does looking at a phased image on the television screen: there were two distinct persons superimposed on each other, but it was very hard to sort out who was what.
>
> (Khan 1971: 236, cited by J.M. Davies 1996: 553)

Davies then poses some of the questions which currently preoccupy the analytic world, on which research from the area of neuroscience may shed some small light. She asks: 'is self integrated, singular, internally coherent, structured linearly upon the accruing bedrock of phase specific developmental crises?' (Davies 1996: 553). And later; 'is the very notion of an integrated internal world a necessary illusion, a metaphoric, functional conduit, providing safe passage across more intrinsically discordant aspects of internalised but essentially irreconcilable aspects of self-other experience?' (Davies 1996: 553). She refers to William James's concept of the mind as 'a confederation of psychic entities' (Taylor 1982: 35, cited in Davies 1996: 553) and goes on to suggest that the extremes of self-organization seen in patients who suffer from multiplicity may in fact 'represent the extreme manifestation of what is perhaps a more accurate rendering of the internal structure of mind' (Davies 1996: 554).

The associative self

As LeDoux has reminded us

> different components of the self reflect the operation of different brain systems ... while explicit memory is mediated by a single system, there are a variety of brain systems that store information implicitly, allowing for many aspects of the self to coexist.
>
> (LeDoux 2002: 31)

The early self schemas proposed by the attachment theorists are the scaffolding for the mind, built by the earliest experiences of relating that are held in implicit memory, and may be more or less coherent depending on the coherence of the child's early experience. Devinsky reminds us that 'the right cerebral hemisphere dominates our awareness of physical and emotional self . . . and a primordial sense of self' (Devinsky 2000: 69). Siegel comments: 'Human connections shape the neural connections from which the mind emerges' (Siegel 1999: 2). Jacques (see Chapter 1), whose early experience was one of coherence and continuity of warm, empathic caretaking, has become a young man with a clear and coherent sense of who he is. He is able to function effectively in many different aspects of being and relating. Bromberg explains

> the shifting configuration of self-states that we call self-hood . . . in order to function optimally, must be at once fluid and robust . . . [this] developmental achievement . . . depends . . . on how well the capacity for affect-regulation and affective competency has been achieved.
>
> (Bromberg 2000: 688)

Schore comments:

> The security of the attachment bond is directly related to
> the developmental neurobiological tenet that optimal secure
> attachment experiences facilitate the experience-dependent
> maturation of a right-lateralised affect regulatory system.
>
> (Schore, in press)

The dissociative self

Our understanding of attachment theory and trauma theory and the
processes of dissociation has come out of growing awareness and
understanding of patients who, rather than, as Redfearn (1985)
suggests, move seamlessly between different aspects of themselves
while retaining a sense of a core self 'I', instead may struggle to
retain a sense of coherence when faced with that which triggers
implicit memory of early psychically painful experience. It has led
Davies to suggest that 'the unconscious structure of mind is fundamentally dissociative rather than repressive in nature' (Davies 1996:
564). I would suggest that the initial state of the brain is unassoci-
ated rather than dissociative, that in health the natural impetus is
towards ever-increasing connectivity resulting in associated states
of mind, giving rise to varied but interlinked self-states. Some
repression of that which enters mind but is rejected occurs. I understand what Davies describes to be the structure of mind rather to
be the structure of the traumatized mind. Schore (2005) notes
that attachment trauma 'induces an enduring impairment of what
Emde (1983) terms the "affective core", the primordial central
integrating structure of the nascent self [and reminds us that] Joseph
(1992) localizes this core system in the right brain and the limbic
system' (Schore 2005, in press). Davies describes that which had to
be dissociated as

> dyadic experiences which are not yet assimilable [and suggests
> that metaphorically they roam] the mind in a hungry search for
> vulnerable moments, using their magnetic charge to disrupt
> the established order and to pull the patient into all forms of
> mystifying, inexplicable enactment.
>
> (Davies 1996: 563)

Holly

Holly (whose dream images are described in Chapter 8) brought a final image (see Plate 3) which seemed to picture her early experience of her mother, but it also described her experience of me at a difficult moment in the transference in the previous day's session, which had precipitated entry into the painful kind of self-state that Davies describes as an unformulated dyadic representation (Davies 1996: 563). After we had looked at this last image together for a while my patient became able to say:

> No brain-clouds, blue sky, no storm just empty space.
> Tight band, locked into position, a belt that beats, stopping any movement between senses and mind. Squeezing, terrible headache.
> Heavy lock in front of my eyes, weighing me down, bumping and banging until I feel mad.
> No nose or mouth. Nothing can be taken in, no food, no air, no life. There is no thoughts to speak, no way of speaking.
> Ears bleeding, the scrambled insides pouring out. Stomach rising to find an opening, blocking sound, just the rush of pain that sits at the core.
> The bullets, words, keep their continuous screaming entry, liquefying everything. No particles are left.

Jung describes how the traumatic complex 'forces itself tyrannically upon the conscious mind. The explosion of affect is a complete invasion of the individual. It pounces upon him like an enemy or a wild animal' (Jung 1928: para. 267). Kalsched (1999) makes a pertinent comment when he observes that

> the reason Jung's notion of the psyche's 'inner persons' is so important is that it ... led to his technique of working with dream and fantasy products on the subjective level: that is, each image is taken as part of the self.
>
> (Kalsched 1999: 467)

I would go so far as to suggest that each image represents one of the many self-states that go to make up the multifaceted relational self.

One patient, towards the end of her analysis, sought to articulate to me her experience of changing self-states, saying:

> I wasn't aware when it was a different aspect of me. At the time I was in it that state would seem all that there was, the competent lawyer that was my coping self vanished, there was only the seemingly limitless and unending pain of the hurt child state.

Solomon warns that 'change only occurs perilously. And . . . that, as much as there are positive forces that seek to move the psyche into the future, there are also powerful retrograde forces that seek to prevent such movement' (Solomon 1998: 226). Such patients arrive in the consulting-room appearing able to cope but they manage at a price, often using large amounts of energy to keep knowledge of the unassimilated self-states at bay. For example, Davies and Frawley (1994) emphasize the ability of the patient who has experienced childhood sexual abuse to 'painstakingly erect the semblance of a functioning, adaptive interpersonally related self around the screaming core of a wounded and abandoned child' (Davies and Frawley 1994: 67). They describe this child aspect of the patient as a 'fully developed dissociated, rather primitively organised alternative self' (Davies and Frawley 1994: 67). They suggest that with such clients the analyst must be aware of both the coping adult self and the hidden abused child in the patient who presents for therapy.

Kalsched (1996) has also described a similar process; he suggests that part of the patient grows up too soon and develops into a coping false self, much as Winnicott suggested, and part of the patient remains too young; experienced as 'the child', the true self remains hidden deep within the personality. He argues that recall of actual abuse stimulates archetypal images and notes that a powerful protector/persecutor figure (much like a harsh super-ego) is often encountered within the structure of the personality who actively seeks to guard the 'imperishable spirit', the true self, from annihilation, even long after the danger is past. I understand these images as attempts of the mind to represent those experiences that have remained encapsulated in the emotional brain.

Sophie

One patient, Sophie, already introduced to the reader on page 51, in the first years of her analysis, painted a series of pictures which illustrated the symbolic emergence of self, as ways of being, born of trauma, emerged and were transformed through experience in the analytic dyad. The early ones showed her dawning sense of her damaged inner being that had occurred through her relation to her mother, and the change and gradual emergence of herself as her experience of inner well-being changed through her experience in the analytic relationship. These pictures were produced at home during the analysis and brought occasionally to a session. The first picture (see Plate 4) vividly described the patient's defended self at the beginning of the analysis, deeply buried in a sarcophagus-like structure, the walls of which were constructed out of her earliest experiences of relationship. The second and the third (see Plates 5 and 6) showed more clearly the way that defended state had come about, and the fourth and fifth (see Plates 7 and 8) the emergence of the self as the analysis enabled the defences to be relinquished and released a new energy for living. The pictures were produced in the first four years of a six-year analysis. Two years later, Sophie painted one further picture (Plate 9); for discussion of this, see pp. 185–6.

Sophie, an artist, who I saw four times weekly for five years, was in her late thirties when she sought help because she had suddenly become unable to work or take care of her family, wishing only to retreat to bed. By the time she came to see me she had been off work for three months. She was depressed, unable to sleep and frightened by what was happening to her. She had two children, a daughter aged 9 years and a son who was 14 years old when she came into analysis. In her early twenties her first child, a son, had been stillborn. His funeral had been held without her knowledge while she was still in hospital. She felt that she had never been able to complete her grieving for him. A counsellor who she had seen for several months when she first became ill referred Sophie to me. She had formed a very intense, possessive transference to him. He felt out of his depth and referred her on to me. She came to analysis because she was frightened by her illness but inevitably started the analysis with a strong negative transference. I was not the ideal and idealized male counsellor; rather I was an uncomfortably close reminder of her denying and depriving mother.

The third girl in a family where a son was longed for, Sophie's history is that of early relational trauma, followed by a seemingly isolated incident of childhood sexual abuse. Her mother had felt that the third child was bound to be a boy. She had a difficult labour and when Sophie was born she would not even look at her. The nanny looked after her and her father named her. Her mother was unable to breastfeed Sophie. At 2 weeks old she was hospitalized without her mother. She is uncertain for how long. When she was a child her mother often said: 'You were the worst, you were ill and you should have been a boy'. She felt that she could never please her mother because she was neither interested in feminine things like her eldest sister nor very attractive like her middle sister, rather she liked to get out into the countryside or to paint. Her mother considered both a waste of time for a girl. Sophie's paintings have documented shifts in her inner world during the analysis. Not surprisingly she brought none for the first six months and then brought the first. She produced it very hesitantly.

In the analysis Sophie's mother came across as unhappy and bitter. Sophie experienced her as cold, blaming and uncaring. When as a child Sophie was admitted to hospital after a bad fall from her bicycle, her mother did not come to visit her for several days and when she came, Sophie remembered her first words as, 'Well what have you managed to do now?', a refrain repeated throughout her childhood. Sophie told me that the only moment she felt she had pleased her mother was when she announced her engagement to a naval officer, seemingly a rather selfish only son, the apple of his mother's eye. The marriage had become sterile before the analysis began and the couple separated during the analysis. Sophie felt that the next two pictures showed her internalized relationships as a series of cogs interacting with one another. In telling me about these paintings Sophie described her mother as the bad cog mother and we acknowledged that it was how she sometimes experienced me in the transference, although she sought to keep me as an idealized good mother. She felt that her mother's cog had damaged her cogs and had thus made it difficult for her to get along with others; she felt that her experience of her mother as the tearing, hurting, destroying mother was lodged inside her, affecting the way she encountered and reacted to others.

Sophie had turned to her father for closeness and until his son was born, when she was 12 years old, he had treated her as the son he longed for and took her around the estate with him. She had longed to be a boy so that she might inherit the estate that she loved so much; indeed until her brother was born, she enjoyed this special relationship with her father and secretly cherished a dream that somehow it might be possible for her to inherit the estate.

In the third picture the mother's cog is seen as a wheel with spikes whirling round and tearing into the flesh of Sophie's hand. With negative feelings so firmly and understandably experienced in relation to her mother, an important part of the work has been to help Sophie to understand her own destructive impulses. It has been difficult to approach the fantasies of her own destructiveness which were apparent in her feelings about the death of her son and were manifest in her inability to care for her own children at the time of her breakdown, which occurred when her daughter reached the age she had been when she experienced a sexually abusive encounter. In her professional life she is strongly identified with the rescuer working skilfully with and on behalf of vulnerable children.

About a year into the analysis Sophie recounted abuse by the 20-year-old gardener on the estate when she was 8 years old. He had enticed her into the garden-shed telling her he had a surprise, a new pet for her. He had shut the door. She remembered the dense quality of the darkness. She described how he had begun to touch her and had tried to force her to touch him, pretending that what she touched was the new pet. She managed to wriggle away and to escape. Afterwards she ran away and hid; she did not feel able to tell anyone. Sophie never entirely forgot the abuse she experienced, but nevertheless managed to put it out of mind until her daughter became the age that she was when the abuse occurred. It was then that she became ill and sought treatment for depression. The memory of the abuse only came directly to mind in the consulting-room when, in a session some three years into the analysis, somewhere outside, a door suddenly banged shut at a tense moment in the transference and reminded her of the clanging shut of the garden-shed door when the abuse took place.

Prior to this Sophie's happy times as a child had been wandering around the estate, and helping with the animals; later she turned more to drawing and painting. Her mother disapproved of all of these activities, but her father encouraged her love of animals, giving her her own flock of sheep to care for. His attitude to her changed as soon as her brother became old enough to walk the farm with him. She had a special walk along a lane that was part of their land. Once she imagined that as she walked there alone she met an ET type character from outer space. He saw inside her and said: 'We are the same you and I, we look one way on the outside but our real self inside is very different'. Although Sophie had to conform outwardly it seems that she never entirely lost awareness of her inner truth. Her adaptive self appears to have been just that, rather than an entirely false self that left no room for awareness of inner truth.

As the analysis continued, so gradually her paintings began to show a softening of the protective shell to allow the gradual emergence of the true self. Four years into the analysis, Sophie painted what appeared to be the last picture in the series (Plate 8), which I came to understand as revealing the gradual emergence of the true self. Sophie spent another four years consolidating the experience portrayed in the pictures. Now she would describe herself as much happier. She is engaged in a meaningful relationship, she has a close relationship with her children and has recently gained promotion at work. She continues to work with vulnerable children but her approach to the task is less heroic.

A trauma patient's early experience causes the self to retreat, hidden from the world by protective defences. Analytic work that encompasses relational as well as interpretive agents of change can bring about the integration of the activity of the hemispheres of the mind-brain that then permits the self to emerge more fully through the process of individuation.

Parallel selves

Others, whose experience before the age of 6 years may have been even more disruptive, profoundly disorienting at best or severely abusive at worst, experience several parallel selves living parallel lives in the same body, often entirely unaware of one another, 'a linear series of separate lives, sequentially lived' (Davies 1996: 566). Sinason (2002) movingly describes her dawning awareness of multiplicity in one of her adult patients and interestingly both Sinason (2002: 133–4) and Goodwin (2002: 139–48) turn to the use of fairy tale to enhance their understanding of dissociative identity disorder. The vertical splits that result from trauma may be seen as an extreme form of the subpersonalities, posited by Redfearn (1985) and linked by him with archetypal images; this may go part way to explain why fairy tales come so readily to mind as the analyst tries to absorb such difficult states of mind.

Mollon (1996) has written in detail about the nature of dissociated identity syndrome from a psychoanalytic viewpoint. It is outside of the scope of this book to explore these ideas in depth but the research into the brain activity described by Reinders et al. (2003) in such patients when they experience different self-states is of crucial importance to our understanding of the way in which the contribution of contemporary neuroscience can help to clarify and to confirm understanding of such complex states that we seek to diagnose and to treat in the consulting-room.

One brain, two selves, or many selves

Reinders et al. (2003) explain that, in order to explore the possibility of one human brain being able to initiate (at least) two autobiographical selves, PET scanning took place while previously prepared scripts were recorded by the therapist in a non-emotive voice. 'The anatomical localization of self-awareness and the brain mechanisms involved in consciousness were investigated by functional neuroimaging different emotional mental states of core consciousness in patients with Multiple Personality Disorder' (Reinders et al. 2003: 2119).

The researchers were able to choose eleven female patients who, as a result of therapy, had become able 'to perform self-initiated and self-controlled switches' (Reinders et al. 2003: 2120) between one of their (what the researchers termed) 'neutral' or 'apparently normal' personality states and one of their 'traumatic' or 'emotional' personality states. The Traumatic Personality State (TPS) of the patient was identified as being able to store a traumatic memory and able to acknowledge that its reactivation affected them emotionally while the Neutral Personality State (NPS) was reported to

be emotionally unresponsive to that memory and had no awareness of having been exposed to that event (Reinders et al. 2003: 2120).
The results demonstrated that

> these patients have state-dependent access to autobiographical affective memories and thus different autobiographical selves. The existence of different regional cerebral blood flow patterns for different senses of self [were observed and explicit roles noted for] the MPFC (medial prefrontal cortex) and the posterior associative cortices in the representation of these different states in consciousness.
>
> (Reinders et al. 2003: 2124)

The right MPFC, thought to play a crucial role in the representation of the self concept, was significantly deactivated when the neutral personality 'listened to the trauma script'. Changes in visual association area and other related areas

> reflect an inability of NPS to ingrate visual and somatosensory information. This 'blocking' of trauma-related information prevents further emotional processing, which reflects the defense system, as applied by DID patients, to enable them to function in daily life.
>
> (Reinders et al. 2003: 2122)

Here I think the researchers are describing the physiological underpinning of an extreme form of what Fordham (1976) identified as the defences of the self. Areas which play a role in regulating emotional and behavioural reaction to pain were activated when the TPS listened to the trauma script but not when the autonomic nervous system heard the same script. The researchers conclude: 'activation in these areas in TPS, as compared to NPS, in reaction to the trauma-related script, thus shows emotional and behavioural dissociation in DID patients' (Reinders et al. 2003: 2123).

The emergent self

How then is a sense of self created within the brain? Panksepp considers this to be 'one of the foremost problems of neuroscience' (Panksepp 2003: 199). He proposes that the experience of emotional feelings arises from the interaction of the variety of emotional networks in the brain with areas in the medial strata of the brain (anterior cingulate, insular and frontal cortices, in turn connected to structures such as the periaqueductal grey). Having a sense of self is dependent on consciousness but how does consciousness come about? How do the various elements of experience merge and then emerge to give us that moment by moment awareness out of which emerges a sense of self, a sense of what it is to be me. Understanding of the self in terms of complex, shifting self-states is congruent with the view of self-consciousness as multi-track, advocated by philosophers such as O'Brien and Opie (2003) who turn to the work of some neuroscientists for evidence to support this view. For example they cite the work of Zeki and Bartels (1998) concerning visual processing, which has indicated that when a particular scene is presented, all aspects of the scene are not perceived simultaneously. This research suggests rather that colour is perceived first, followed by orientation, and only after that is motion perceived (Zeki and Bartels 1998, cited in O'Brien and Opie 2003: 115). As a result of their experimental work Zeki and Bartels conclude that there are 'multiple visual micro-consciousnesses which are asynchronous with respect to each other' (Zeki and Bartels 1998: 1584, cited in O'Brien and Opie 2003: 116). O'Brien and Opie summarize:

> With this hypothesis goes a view about the neural basis of self, namely, that it depends on many distinct centres of representation within the brain; from the cortical regions associated with somatotopic body-mapping and action-mapping, through regions that function to distinguish between self-initiated and externally caused events, up to regions such as the prefrontal cortex that play a crucial role in organising behaviour.
> (O'Brien and Opie 2003: 117)

This being the case, they go on to explore how a sense of being a single self might emerge from the multiplicity of consciousness. They conclude that 'a sense of self emerges when the multiple tracks of self-directed experience produced by the brain are sufficiently *representationally coherent*' (O'Brien and Opie 2003: 117, italics in original), and suggest that one of the neural structures previously thought to produce consciousness *per se* may actually be better construed as a 'self-maker' rather than a 'conscious-maker'. Schore suggests that there are dual representations of the self, the left hemisphere dealing with verbal self-description, one might consider as 'the explicit self' while the right hemisphere deals with 'the affective sense of self' (Schore 2005 in press). It seems to me that one might characterize that which arises from the left hemisphere as 'the explicit self', and that which arises from the right one might term 'the implicit self.'

In the following clinical material I seek to show the developing self as experienced in a series of dreams that marked pivotal points in an analysis. The self system is understood as a hierarchical system developing from the lower subcortical processing structures, through the early dyadic experience, to the higher, more complex, fine-detailed cortical structures, enabling reflective function and orbitofrontal, inhibitory control. The pivotal points in this analysis were each announced by a dream about the attachment relationship. I have concentrated on these in order to show the evolution of the core, germinal aspects of the self and the change from insecure to secure attachment occurring in the growth-facilitating environment of the attuned transference/countertransference relationship. This case material appeared in the *Journal of Analytical Psychology* in February 2004.

Mark

When I opened the door to Mark for the first time, he stood there, looked long at me, then enunciated his name very clearly. I had a feeling that an event of significance had occurred. It was his concern about his stutter and especially the way it affected his ability to say his name that brought him into treatment. Eventually I came to appreciate the significance that the conflict over saying his name might have in his struggle for separateness and a sense of his own identity.

Mark, who was in his late twenties, was the only child of a narcissistic, alcoholic mother who found it difficult to permit him any degree of separateness. He was kept in nappies until he was 4 years old. His cot had cushions around it because he was inclined to head banging. He was not allowed to play with other children and does not remember having toys or games. Rather he was his mother's companion, just allowed to watch as she worked around the house. Each night when he came home from school he had to eat 'a huge dinner' as soon as he came home, in spite of the school lunch he had already eaten and the evening meal she provided later. Each night at bedtime she exhorted him that they should dream the same dream. He felt that he did everything late: he did not read until he was 11. His main memory of childhood is of being in what might be described as an autistic state, in which he rocked endlessly, sometimes singing as he did so. His stutter seems to have acted as a barrier to protect the self from being overwhelmed by the mother. At the same time it protected both from knowing of his hatred and guilt. If he could have spoken freely what might he have said to a mother such as his?

Mark's mother made several suicide attempts during his childhood and was compulsorily hospitalized at least once. His father, denigrated by his wife, was the outsider in the family triangle, and he looked to Mark to be the caretaking adult for the baby mother. His father turned to Mark for help when she locked herself in the kitchen with the gas on, or in the bathroom with her wrists slashed. Thus attempts to relate to the father led not to the outside world but inexorably back to mother. He became tearful, depressed and school phobic. He was put on Valium, which he took throughout his teens. His mother died of the effects of alcoholism when he was 21 years old.

First phase of analysis: dreams arising from an insecure, disorganized attachment and subcortical, amygdala-driven states of fear and dread

Dream 1

He came downstairs in a house where he had lived as a child; he went into a room and saw *his mother* in a corner with *her face slashed*.

Dream 2

He was inside a room and seeking to protect a young boy from awful danger outside. He locked the door but it was no good, a large and menacing woman managed to get into the room. As she came towards him *he looked into her face and was filled with dread*.

These early dreams outlined to me in stark detail just what the internal working model of the attachment relationship might be like for my patient, bearing in mind what a potent stimulus the mother's face is for the developing infant. Mark told me the dreams as if in a frozen state of hypo-arousal, entirely without affect. I, too, at first felt nothing, and then I was more able to become aware of my feelings and the terrifying nature of the images. As I began to feel afraid, so Mark began to talk, for the first time, about the detail of one of his mother's suicide attempts that occurred when he was 8 years old. Mark recounted:

> She locked herself in the kitchen with the gas on. Dad came up to my bedroom and asked whether I thought I could get her out. We went downstairs. I tried to persuade her, I was crying and all that. She wouldn't come out.

For a moment the room was full of feeling. I felt I was listening to a young boy, needing to dismiss his tears and the pain they repre-sented. I was also aware of the very small baby, who had reached the stage of frantic distress that then leads to the dissociative defence of detachment from the unbearable situation, 'the escape where there is no escape'. He went on to tell of his grandmother's and mother's deaths. He said: 'I felt at a distance from it all. I didn't feel anything'. I commented: 'Perhaps Mum was the only one who was allowed to have strong feelings?' 'Yes, that's how it was', Mark concluded. Because of his mother's difficulties Mark did have some sense of a damaged mother, the damaging mother of the second dream was much less accessible to consciousness. Rather there was a timeless, overwhelming feeling to the way he described her. Boundaries seemed non-existent and it was as if I became the mother from whom his infant brain had imprinted such dysregulated states of fear and terror.

The way this particular session developed illustrates the way in which the emergence of a dream may carry elements of actual trau-matic experience, will certainly reflect the patient's internal world and will indicate the elements of the patient's internal world that are dominating the transference at the time. It is a matter of fine judge-ment on the part of the analyst as to which of these to pursue at any time. However, the patient lives in the present and it is the present experience within the current dyad that can effect change, thus the particular aspects of past experience that emerge must be understood in relation to current relationship.

Second phase of analysis: dreams that illustrate the beginnings of change and cingulate-driven, dyadic attempts to connect

After the first long break, about ten months into the analysis, there seemed to be a shift and I began to feel that Mark could, at least fleetingly, experience the presence of two minds. On his return he reiterated his hatred of stammering, saying, 'because when I stammer I cease to feel at one with people'. I interpreted his anger and my seeming unreliability. The attack continued until I said, 'You feel as if I am cruel and murderous and that you are the victim. But I also feel that I am being attacked as your no good mother analyst. It feels as if you are the attacker and I am the victim'. In the following session Mark brought a dream:

Dream 3

His mother produced pills that were old and had become poison. She told him this and that they could commit suicide together. They took them and began to feel funny. *They were not able to see each other clearly.* Mark suggested they should go to hospital.

Again his dream refers to the gaze sequence of the mother–infant dyad. Now the dreamer is no longer in a state of terror, but there are still difficulties in the gaze–gaze away sequence that characterizes mother–infant interaction, an essential part of the process of building healthy connectivity in the infant brain. The dream also indicates that the feed this mother offered would lead, not to life, but death. Again the child, not the mother, is the caretaker. However, there is vocalization and with it the hope of connectedness. A further dream followed at this time.

Dream 4

He was serving drinks at a sherry party in the hospital where he worked. His mother was shut away in an institution. He wondered, 'Should we invite her?' Someone said, 'No, if she's shut away leave her there'.

Mark recounted this dream with difficulty, hampered by the stammer that the experience of a separate, emergent self evoked. He recounted a recent fantasy of being a conductor controlling an orchestra. I said, 'I think you want to be able to control me and the sounds I make, maybe even silence me altogether?' For a moment the hatred was out in the open, then he laughed and said, 'That was an underhand way to do it'. At this time he recalled his first memory of hostility towards his mother, when he had sought to protect his adopted younger brother from her attack. The emergence of this material began to suggest a growing capacity to protect and mother the child within.

Final phase of analysis: dreams indicating the development of secure attachment and higher, more complex cortical development, characterized by the emergence of reflective function and orbitofrontal inhibitory control

After about two years of analysis Mark brought the final dream of the sequence

> Dream 5
>
> I dreamed of my mother. She was dead. She seemed to be having something drawn off. It seemed as if she had a scrotum or a womb, and it was something from there . . . Maybe I was doing it. I don't think so but maybe I was because I don't remember anyone else being there . . . a sort of nothingness, maybe like a mortuary. She wasn't like her. *Her face didn't look like her, her hair was messy, she was skinny, there were no breasts* . . . She was dead but *it was something I'd got to do before I could get free of her.* I kept trying to hold onto her but she was sort of squashy and I couldn't.

This dream seemed to indicate that enough work had been done in the therapeutic dyad for the dreamer to become able to reflect about how he perceived his mother and his relation to her. I asked, 'Do you feel there is anything you have to do in relation to your dead mother?' He replied, 'Well, I feel I have to get free of her. I have to get my life separate from her'. He continued, 'You know the worst was I didn't know what to do with her. I couldn't find anywhere suitable to put her so I couldn't let her go'. He began to sound insecure and frightened. After a while I said, 'I think it's what to do with the Mum inside you that you find so difficult and frightening . . . it's how you've felt here sometimes. You once said to me, "I feel disloyal if I look at how things were with Mum, where does that put her?"'

By the end of this period of the analysis Mark was much more consistently able to have a sense of being alone yet contained. My sense of the birth of the self was reflected in a memory he produced at this time of a childhood solitary cycle ride, something his mother did not allow. He had come upon an orchard in full bloom. He crossed a stile and walked there among the trees, sensing the beauty and mystery of him and the orchard.

How did Mark's stutter arise? What did it signify in relation to his developing self? Sound-making communication begins as an entirely emotional experience, located in the amygdala. Schore (1994) stresses that one-word speech arises out of affective interchanges with the mother that are imprinted in the right hemisphere. He comments: 'The child's name is typically the first emotion word that the child learns' (Schore 1994: 488). I suggest that Mark's stutter was symptomatic of him getting 'stuck' in the processes of separation, because of his need to remain fused with his mother as a response to early relational trauma. It resulted in his inability to internalize the ordinary dialogue of a gradually separating infant and mother and to develop 'inner-talk', that is, thought. Speculatively one might also wonder whether Mark's damaging early experience, encoded in his right brain, may have kept his attempts at sound making partially located there also.

In his second dream Mark sought to protect a young child from a dangerous, engulfing, witch-like mother. His stutter may be understood symbolically, as a protective barrier, a very particular kind of false, adaptive self that sought to preserve the integrity of the true self until better times. It kept him isolated and 'safe', permitting only a false self to be seen, keeping his unique, individual self well hidden. His analysis with its gradual and repeated deintegratory and reintegratory experiences of safe separateness with me enabled the purposeful unfolding of the Primal Self in relation to another. Mark commented in his final session: 'Now, I barely think of my stutter, I wonder more what people will think of me'.

Conclusion

Looking at the research findings it seems to me that, although the predisposition to develop a sense of self is hard-wired from the beginning, the essence of the individual self that emerges is defined by the earliest experience of relationships that enable patterns of neural connectivity to establish in the brain. These relationships become stored in implicit memory, determining our most fundamental ways of being and relating and may in health be experienced as self-states through which we move seamlessly as occasion and inner urge demand. For the analyst awareness of that patterning is crucial; that awareness is achieved through both transference and countertransference. Thus the new experience of relating in the analytic dyad is fundamental to the successful outcome of the therapy. It is this new experience of relating, aided by left brain insight arising out of interpretation, that enables a more coherent sense of self.

Postscript

What happens within oneself when one integrates previously
unconscious contents with consciousness is something which can
scarcely be described in words. It can only be experienced. It is a
subjective affair quite beyond discussion; we have a particular
feeling about ourselves, about the way we are, and that is a fact
which it is neither possible nor meaningful to doubt. Similarly, we
convey a particular feeling to others.

(Jung 1962: 318)

Contemporary neuroscience has much to offer the contemporary
Jungian analyst who seeks to reframe their thinking in response to
contemporary scientific thought. Ehrlich (2003), in his discussion of
working at the frontier, suggests that when we consider the findings
of bio-physiology we may find that we develop a dual vision of man:
man as 'the neuronal man [and man as] the discerning subject'
(Ehrlich 2003: 236). I would add that, nevertheless, it must be a
dual vision that frees itself of the old Cartesian split, for both the
neuronal man and the discerning subject are one and indissoluble, a
human mind-brain-body being. Ehrlich suggests that depth psychology has thrived on just such seemingly irreconcilable tensions
since its inception, arguing that 'psychoanalysis is the study of man
that makes the strange and the alien inherent within the subject its
vehicle, method and yield' (Ehrlich 2003: 236). As I have read and
discussed with colleagues, I have come to value increasingly the
opportunities that are now available to us to explore new and at
first strange, even alien-seeming to some, territory in order to gain a
better appreciation of the nature of the terrain of our analytic
homeland.

First, it has become clear to me that with many patients our task is to help them to come to terms with damaging early relational trauma, laid down in implicit, amygdaloidal, emotional memory, revealed in feelings of abandonment, terror and dread. Thoughtful attention to sympathetic nervous system based experiences of arousal permits modulation by the analyst's sensitive response, which at the same time helps the patient to stay engaged with the point of pain. In any session a traumatized patient may experience rapidly alternating states of sympathetic nervous system arousal and parasympathetic nervous system damping down to the point of helpless, numb withdrawal. The analyst's task is often to help these patients to experience a middle place very different to the extremes of emotional experience and pain of abandonment to which early and continuing trauma exposed them. In the session it means neither ignoring the mounting level of distress, nor reassuring, but rather taking care to keep the degree of distress at a manageable level, while returning to the point of pain.

Second, research into affective neuroscience provides insights concerning the effects of trauma on the brain. Perry et al. (1995) note that

> Ultimately, it is the human brain that processes and internalises traumatic (and therapeutic) experiences. It is the brain that mediates all emotional, cognitive, behavioral, social, and physiological functioning. It is the human brain from which the human mind arises and within that mind resides our humanity. Understanding the organisation, function, and development of the human brain, and brain-mediated responses to threat, provides the keys to understanding.
>
> (Perry et al. 1995: 273)

If profound dissociative defences are to be undone in those for whom poor early experience with the primary care-giver has resulted in trauma, awareness of the science of loss and recovery of memory and right brain engagement of the therapist with right brain aspects of the patient in therapy are essential. Only alongside such affective encounters does it become possible for the left brain to fully process traumatic experience.

Third, I would suggest that insights from neuroscience under-line what research into the effectiveness of psychotherapy has generally shown to be true: that the foundation for 'coming into mind' must be a secure attachment to the analyst. This allows the patient to begin to venture confidently to explore difference and to have the repeated experiences of safe separateness. These in turn permit awareness of one's own mind in relation to another mind, the only true basis for genuine intimacy. Mitrani (2001), in her exploration of the notion of the second skin (Bick 1968; Symington 1985; Anzieu 1989), suspects that an

> *attitude of extreme compliance* that, while simulating improvement, merely signals the development of a new and more subtle version of the second skin; one that is patterned on the personality and theories of the analyst and is therefore 'acceptable' to him.
>
> (Mitrani 2001: 5, italics in original)

Such defensive attempts at illusory rather than genuine intimacy may occur as the patient seeks to protect the therapy from inner destructive rage. A patient may long to experience oneness or non-difference with the analyst, for it is perceived as the only safe way of being with another. Fonagy (1991) comments:

> Individuals whose primary objects are unloving and cruel may find contemplation of the contents of the mind of the object unbearable. Overwhelmed by intolerable aggression from within and without, the individual desperately seeks comfort in a regressive fusion with the object, 'a rescuing parent'.
>
> (Fonagy 1991: 649)

Some of the difficulties that arise in such therapies come about because the analyst allows just such an illusion of oneness to persist for too long. The experience of pseudo-togetherness in place of genuine intimacy will evoke the earlier relational trauma and may cause the patient to despair. Rather, what is required is an experience of safe separateness that can call forth change from within.

Fourth, knowledge of the developing mind-brain in the early years, and again in adolescence, enables us to appreciate the mind-brain underpinning of attachment and the significance of the critical part played by the impact of early negative experience on the developing life of the individual child, and ultimately on the life of our society. Perry et al. note that 'different events at different times in

the life of an individual are likely to result in a different combination of adaptive responses' (Perry et al. 1995: 286). The process of
establishing an adequate affective bond between child and primary
care-giver enables first of all, regulation of affect by the mother, and
then by the age of about 18 months, the possibility of self-regulation
begins to develop. Carvalho (2002) emphasizes the importance of
successful negotiation of this process, which, with Schore (1994),
he associates with the mother's mind enabling the infant's mind,
her right orbitofrontal cortex standing proxy for her infant's until
it is ready to come on line (Carvalho 2002: 159). If it fails he
suggests that both the infant and later the adult 'is prey to overwhelming and often disorganised and disorganising affects together
often with autonomic discharge, and/or with other somatic manifestation . . . because mind is overwhelmed' (Carvalho 2002: 157).
Carvalho goes on to argue that the only other alternative is that,
rather than thought becoming trapped in the symptom, only
thought prevails, and the patient becomes 'very rationalistic and
divorced from feeling, emotion and bodily states' (Carvalho 2002:
157). I would add that, along the continuum of self-experience
moving towards the self-experiences associated with dissociative
identity disorder, patients may move from the extreme of one state
to the extreme of the other as alternating subjectivities are
experienced.

Siegel notes that one of the significant findings to emerge from
attachment research is that of the presence of a group of adults
characterised as the 'earned secure' (Siegel 2003: 16). As mind
changes through interaction with the therapist, acting in the role of
a secondary care-giver, so the nature of poor early attachment, the
response to early trauma can change. Therapy offers the possibility
of the emergence of this new kind of attachment. I would actually
characterize the desired new outcome as 'learned secure', rather
than 'earned secure'. 'Earned secure' has some of the negative over-
tones of the kind of experience that abused children may encounter
in placement in foster families. Having to earn attachment is
unlikely to produce a secure attachment. As analysts know to their
cost, this kind of experience in the therapy room may well foster a
profound negative transference in which the analyst becomes
experienced as the abusive other and the 'placement' (to continue
the analogy with fostering) may break down irretrievably. Affective
neuroscience is encouraging in that the emphasis on plasticity, with
its possibility of the remaking of mind, means that the empathetic

analyst may be experienced in a new way, leading to change in the very nature of basic attachment, meriting a new category of attachment, that of 'learned secure'.

Fifth, the role of empathy in analysis has often been devalued, indeed even seen as a distraction or a defensive manoeuvre engineered by the patient to avoid the real work, the talking-cure. However, I believe that Fordham (1957) had the right of it when he described the need for the analyst to be open to deintegrative processes within in order to put at the patient's disposal spontaneity of relating coming from deep within the analyst. I quote:

> There are two ways of behaving: (1) trying to isolate oneself from the patient by being as integrated as possible and (2) relinquishing this attitude and simply listening to and watching the patient to hear and see what comes out of the self in relation to the patient's activities and then reacting. This would appear to involve deintegrating; it is as if what is put at the disposal of patients are parts of the analyst which are spontaneously responding to the patient in the way that he needs.
>
> (Fordham 1957: 97)

I believe the insights brought to the Jungian world by Fordham blend seamlessly with the developmental neuroscience of Schore, Stern and Siegel, who have examined the effect of early relational experience on the developing brain-mind. Such insights make devaluation of a strongly relational approach to therapy a position that is now virtually untenable. Solms and Turnbull (2002) describe the way in which the motor neurons in a monkey which merely watches another monkey behave in a particular way mirror the characteristic pattern being fired in the motor cortex of the active monkey. They go on to suggest that further research may reveal this as the basis for empathy and the explanation of how children internalize the behaviour of their parents (Solms and Turnbull 2002: 282). It might be just this process that underpins the therapeutic process in the dyad in the consulting-room, as well as forming the basis for some of the damaging countertransference reactions that beset such work. Knox observes that

> as therapists we cannot be merely scientific observers of our patients' mental processes but must also allow ourselves to be drawn in and sometimes taken over emotionally; we must be

able to feel love and hate, sometimes towards and sometimes with or on behalf of our patients.

(Knox 2001: 614)

It is the particular contribution that contemporary neuroscience can make to our understanding of this intuitive process that this book has sought to explore.

Lastly, I believe that very soon the contribution that the new scanning procedures will be able to make to our quest for evidence-based research into clinical practice will be invaluable. Paus (2005) stresses the value of the new scanning procedures, noting that they allow us 'to measure *in vivo* subtle inter-individual differences in brain structure and to assess activity in distinct neural circuits from birth to adulthood' (Paus 2005: 60). Lanius et al. (2004) demonstrate the potential value of such work in their fMRI functional connectivity analysis study of the nature of traumatic memories. Using scanning techniques with two groups of trauma patients, they were able to compare the patterns of connectivity in the group with PTSD symptoms with those without. The study was able to conclude that the differences in brain connectivity between the two groups may account for the non-verbal nature of traumatic memory recall in those with PTSD as opposed to the more verbal pattern of traumatic memory recall in the comparison group (Lanius et al. 2004). However, what cannot be detected by this study is whether those patterns of connectivity preceded the traumatic experience or whether they were the result of it. Using PET scanning Houdé et al. (2001) were able to demonstrate that access to effective deductive logic depends on a right ventromedial prefrontal area devoted to emotion and feeling, thus demonstrating the controlling part that emotion and feeling have in effective thinking (Houdé et al. 2001: 1486–92).

The understanding of the relevance of neuroscience to analytic work is still in its infancy; conclusions as to applications must as yet be tentative. Some things seem clear. The vicissitudes of experience within the analytic dyad facilitate the development of self-regulatory capacity and the emergence of reflective function. The developing emotional connectivity that occurs within the analytic dyad forms the essential psychic scaffolding that enables the complementary work, known traditionally as the talking-cure. The Jungian view of the self is entirely in keeping with the insights that are emerging, as Schore comments:

The centre of psychic life shifts from Freud's *ego*, which he located in the 'speech area on the left hand side' (Freud 1923) and the posterior areas of the verbal left hemisphere, to the highest levels of the right hemisphere, the locus of the bodily based *self* system.

(Schore 2001a: 77, italics in original)

The self-system may manifest itself in many self-states, through which many of us are able to move seamlessly for much of the time; however, work in the consulting-room will involve naming those self-states with some of our patients. Others may require help to deal compassionately with themselves as they experience many selves who clamour for recognition, for yet others increasing integration culminating in the goal Jung described as 'individuation' will be possible.

I have noted with interest the issues raised by others who have written on this subject. Some direct us to the ethical and moral questions that are raised by the abolition of Cartesian dualism, the knowledge that mind and brain are one (Carter 2000; Teicher 2000). These will need to be resolved. Others explore the significance for the consulting-room, for example Pally (2000) closes with the hopefulness inherent in the notion of the flexibility, or plasticity of the human brain. I believe that the emphasis of Solms and Turnbull (2002) perhaps deserves the last word:

In the long term, a comprehensive neuroscience of subjective experience will be developed with or without psychoanalysis. The cooperation of psychoanalysts at this point will surely speed up the process and enrich it immeasurably . . . A radically different psychoanalysis will emerge . . . its claims will be far more securely grounded.

(Solms and Turnbull 2002: 314–15)

As I was writing this postscript, Sophie suddenly found herself painting what was clearly the completion of the series of paintings begun so many years ago (see Chapter 9). She brought it to a session, explaining how it had taken her almost by surprise. It shows not a rigid woman with clenched hands, locked in a sarcophagus of her own persecutory childhood, but a relaxed woman, just about to wake from sleep, under a coverlet decorated with her own personal symbols of hope. There are snowdrops, which early in her analysis were a powerful symbol of the dawning of hope, the beginning of the thaw from the frozen winter of her childhood, and daisies had burgeoned everywhere as she painted, symbols of the coming to flower of a more abundant summertime within (see Plate 9).

I was reminded of Jay's little boy kangaroo (Chapter 6) and Holly's little cream cat (Chapter 8), their personal symbols of hope. From a Jungian viewpoint, I believe insights from contemporary neuroscience may assist us substantially as we travel with our patients on their journeys to deeper self-knowledge, deeper self-fulfilment, the journey that for me is one of 'coming into mind'.

References

Abelin, E. (1971) 'The role of the father in the separation–individuation process', in J.B. McDevitt and C.F. Settlage (eds) *Separation–Individuation*, New York: International Universities Press.

Affeld-Niemeyer, P. (1995) 'Trauma and symbol: instinct and reality perception in therapeutic work with victims of incest', *Journal of Analytical Psychology*, 40 (1): 23–40.

Ainsworth, M.D.S. (1969) 'Object relations, dependence and attachment: a theoretical review of the infant–mother relationship', *Child Development*, 40: 969–1025.

American Psychiatric Association (APA) (1994) *Diagnostic and Statistical Manual of Mental Disorders*, 4th edn (DSM-IV), Washington, DC: APA.

Anzieu, D. (1989) *The Skin Ego*, New Haven, CT: Yale University Press.

Aserinsky, E. and Kleitman, N. (1953) 'Regularly occurring periods of ocular motility and concomitant phenomena during sleep', *Science*, 118: 361–75.

Astor, J. (1988) 'Adolescent states of mind found in patients of different ages seen in analysis', *Journal of Child Psychotherapy*, 14 (1): 67–80.

—— (1998) 'Fordham's developments of Jung in the context of infancy and childhood', in I. Alister and C. Hauke (eds) *Contemporary Jungian Analysis*, London and New York: Routledge.

—— (2005) 'A conversation with Dr Fordham', *Journal of Analytical Psychology*, 50 (1): 9–18; first published in *Journal of Child Psychotherapy* (1988), 14: 3–12.

Beebe, B. and Lachmann, F. (2002) *Infant Research and Adult Treatment: Co-constructing interactions*, Hillsdale, NJ and London: Analytic Press.

Beebe, J. (2005) 'Finding our way in the dark', *Journal of Analytical Psychology*, 50 (1): 91–101.

Bick, E. (1968) 'The experience of the skin in early object relations', *International Journal of Psychoanalysis*, 49: 484–6.

Binet, A., Baldwin, H.H.G. and Baldwin, J.M. (1896) *Alterations of Personality*, New York: D. Appleton.

Bion, W.R. (1977) *Seven Servants*, New York: Aronson.

—— (1990) *Brazilian Lectures*, London: Karnac.

Bovensiepen, G. (2002) 'Symbolic attitude and reverie: problems of symbolisation in children and adolsecents', *Journal of Analytical Psychology*, 47 (2): 241–57.

Bowlby, J. (1969) *Attachment*, London: Pelican.

Brafman, A. (2004) 'Working with adolescents: a pragmatic view', in I. Wise (ed.) *Adolescence*, London and New York: Karnac.

Braun, A. (1999) 'Commentary on the new neuropsychology of sleep', *Neuropsychoanalysis*, 1 (2): 196–201.

Brewin, C.R. and Andrews, B. (1998) 'Recovered memories of trauma: phenomenology and cognitive mechanisms', *Clinical Psychology Review*, 18 (8): 949–70.

Brewin, C.R., Dalgleish, T. and Joseph, S. (1996) 'A dual representation theory of post-traumatic stress disorder', *Psychological Review*, 103: 670–86.

Bromberg, P.M. (2000) 'Bringing in the dreamer: some reflections on dreamwork, surprise and analytic process', *Contemporary Psychoanalysis*, 36: 685–705.

—— (2003) 'One need not be a house to be haunted: on enactment, dissociation, and the dread of "Not-Me" – a case study', *Psychoanalytic Dialogues*, 13 (5): 689–709.

Bronstein, C. (2004) 'Working with suicidal adolescents', in I. Wise (ed.) *Adolescence*, London and New York: Karnac.

Brown, A. (2001) 'Volcanic irruptions', in H. Formaini (ed.) *Landmarks: Papers by Jungian analysts from Australia and New Zealand*, Manuka, Australia: Australian and New Zealand Society of Jungian Analysts.

Bucci, W. (1997) *Psychoanalysis and Cognitive Science: A multiple code theory*, New York and London: Guilford Press.

Buccino, G., Binkofski, F., Fink, G.R., Fadiga, L., Gallese, V., Setz, R.J., Zilles, K., Rizzolatti, G. and Freund, H.J. (2001) 'Action observation activated premotor and parietal areas in a somatotopic manner: an fMRI study', *European Journal of Neuroscience*, 13: 400–4.

Cambray, J. (2005) 'The place of the 17th century in Jung's encounter with China', *Journal of Analytical Psychology*, 50 (2): 191–207.

Cambray, J. and Carter, L. (2004) *Analytical Psychology: Contemporary perspectives in Jungian analysis*, Hove and New York: Brunner-Routledge.

Canli, T. (2004) 'Functional brain-mapping of extraversion and neuroticism: learning from individual differences in emotion processing', *Journal of Personality*, 72 (6): 1105–32.

Carter, R. (2000) *Mapping the Mind*, London: Phoenix.

Carvalho, R. (2002) 'Psychic retreats revisited: binding primitive destructiveness or securing object? A matter of emphasis?', *British Journal of Psychotherapy*, 19 (2): 153–71.

Caspi, A., Sugden, K., Moffitt, T.E., Taylor, A., Craig, I.W., Harrington, H., McClay, J., Mill, J., Martin, J., Braithwaite, A. and Poulton, B. (2003) 'Influence of life stress on depression: moderation by a polymorphism in the 5-HTT gene', *Science*, 301: 386–9.

Chefetz, R.A. (1999) 'Letter to the Editor', *International Journal of Psychoanalysis*, 80 (2): 376–7.

—— (2000) 'Affect dysregulation as a way of life', *Journal of the American Academy of Psychoanalysis*, 28 (2): 289–303.

—— (2005) 'The dissociative self: integrating neuroscience and clinical practice', paper presented at a conference arranged by the International Society for the Study of Dissociation and the Del Amo Hospital, California, February.

Chu, J.A. (1998) *Rebuilding Shattered Lives: The responsible treatment of complex post-traumatic and dissociative disorders*, New York: Wiley.

Chugani, H., Behen, M., Muzik, O., Juhasz, C., Nagi, F. and Chugani, D. (2001) 'Local brain functional activity following early deprivation: a study of Romanian orphans', *Neuroimage*, 14: 1290–301.

Churchland, P.S. (2002) *Brain-Wise: Studies in neurophilosophy*, Cambridge, MA and London: MIT Press.

Clark, G. (2001) 'The animating body: psychoid substance as a mutual experience of psychosomatic disorder', in H. Formaini (ed.) *Landmarks: Papers by Jungian analysts from Australia and New Zealand*, Manuka, Australia: Australian and New Zealand Society of Jungian Analysts.

Clyman, R. (1991) 'The procedural organisation of emotions', in T. Shapiro and R. Emde (eds) *Affect, Psychoanalytic Perspectives*, New York: International Universities Press.

Cole, S., Sumnall, H. and Grob, C. (2002) 'Sorted: Ecstasy', *The Psychologist*, 15 (9): 464–7, 474.

Commins, D.L., Vosmer, G., Virus, R.M., Woolverton, W.L., Schuster, C.R. and Seiden, L.S. (1987) 'Biochemical and histological evidence that methylenedioxymethamphetamine (MDMA) is toxic to neurons in the rat brain', *Journal of Pharmacology and Experimental Therapeutics*, 241: 338–45.

Covington, C. (1995) 'No story, no analysis? The role of narrative in interpretation', *Journal of Analytical Psychology*, 40 (3): 405–17.

Cozolino, L. (2002) *The Neuroscience of Psychotherapy: Building and rebuilding the human brain*, New York and London: W.W. Norton.

Crittenden, D. and Ainsworth, M.D.S. (1989) 'Child maltreatment and attachment theory', in D. Cicchetti and V. Carlson (eds) *Child Maltreatment*, New York: Cambridge University Press.

Croft, R. (2002) 'Ecstasy: "danger" remains', *The Psychologist*, 15 (9): 470–1.

Croft, R.J., Klugman, A., Baldeweg, T. and Gruzelier, J.G.H. (2001) 'Electrophysiological evidence of serotonergic impairment in long-term "ecstasy" users', *American Journal of Psychiatry*, 158: 1687–92.

Culbert-Koehn, J. (1997) 'Don't get stuck in the mother', *Journal of Analytical Psychology*, 42 (1): 99–104.

Damasio, A. (1999) *The Feeling of What Happens: Body, emotion and the making of consciousness*, London: Heinemann.

—— (2004) *Looking for Spinoza: Joy, sorrow, and the feeling brain*, London: Vintage.

Daniels, L. (2000) 'Dreams in pursuit of art', in L. Gamwell (ed.) *Dreams 1900–2000: Science, art and the unconscious mind*, Ithaca, NY: Cornell University Press.

Davies, J.M. (1996) 'Linking the "pre-analytic" with the postclassical: integration, dissociation, and the multiplicity of unconscious process', *Contemporary Psychoanalysis*, 32 (4): 553–76.

Davies, J.M. and Frawley, M.G. (1994) *Treating the Adult Survivor of Childhood Sexual Abuse: A psychoanalytic perspective*, New York: Basic Books.

Davies, M. (2002) 'A few thoughts about the mind, the brain and a child with early deprivation', *Journal of Analytical Psychology*, 47 (3): 421–35.

Decety, J. and Chaminade, T. (2003) 'When the self represents the other: a new cognitive neuroscience view on psychological identification', *Consciousness and Cognition*, 12: 577–96.

Devinsky, O. (2000) 'Right hemisphere dominance', *Epilepsy and Behaviour*, 1: 60–73.

Dmitrieva, J., Chen, C., Greenberger, E. and Gil-Rivas, V. (2004) 'Family relationships and adolescent psychosocial outcomes: converging findings from eastern and western cultures', *Journal of Research on Adolescence*, 14 (4): 425–47.

Eagle, M. (2000) 'The developmental perspectives of attachment and psychoanalytic theory', in P. Goldberg, R. Muir and J. Kerr (eds) *Attachment Theory*, London: Analytic Press.

Edelman, G.M. and Tononi, G. (2000) *Consciousness: How matter becomes imagination*, London: Penguin.

Ehrlich, H.S. (2003) 'Working at the frontier and the use of the analyst: reflections on analytic survival', *International Journal of Psychoanalysis*, 84: 235–47.

Eigen, M. (2001) *Damaged Bonds*, London: Karnac.

Ekstrom, S.R. (2004) 'Freudian, Jungian and cognitive models of the unconscious', *Journal of Analytical Psychology*, 49 (5): 657–82.

—— (2005) 'Response to "The influence of complexes on implicit learning"', *Journal of Analytical Psychology*, 50 (2): 191–3.

Emde, R.N. (1983) 'The pre-representational self and its affective core', *Psychoanalytic Study of the Child*, 38: 165–92.

Everest, P. (1999) 'The multiple self: working with dissociation and trauma', *Journal of Analytical Psychology*, 44 (4): 443–64.

Feldman, B. (2004) 'A skin for the imaginal', *Journal of Analytical Psychology*, 49: 285–311.

Ferro, A. (2005) *Seeds of Illness, Seeds of Recovery: The genesis of suffering and the role of psychoanalysis*, trans. P. Slotkin, New Library of Psychoanalysis series, ed. D. Birksted-Breen, Hove and New York: Brunner-Routledge.

Fonagy, P. (1991) 'Thinking about thinking: some clinical and theoretical considerations in the treatment of a borderline patient', *International Journal of Psychoanalysis*, 76: 639–56.

—— (2000) 'Dreams of borderline patients', in J. Perelberg (ed.) *Dreaming and Thinking*, London: Karnac.

—— (2002) Chairman's comments, Anna Freud Centre Fiftieth Anniversary Conference, School of Oriental and African Studies, London, 2 November.

—— (2003) 'Some complexities in the relation of theory to technique', *Psychoanalytic Quarterly*, 72: 13–47.

—— (2004) 'Psychotherapy meets neuroscience: a more focused future for psychotherapy research', *Psychiatric Bulletin*, 28: 357–9.

Fordham, M. (1957) 'Notes on the transference', in M. Fordham, *New Developments in Analytical Psychology*, London: Routledge.

—— (1969) *Children as Individuals*, London: Hodder and Stoughton.

—— (1976) *The Self and Autism*, London: Heinemann.

—— (1985) *Explorations into the Self*, Library of Analytical Psychology, vol. 7, London: Academic Press.

Fox, H., Parrott, A.C. and Turner, J.J.D. (2001a) 'Ecstasy/MDMA related cognitive deficits: a function of dosage rather than awareness of problems', *Journal of Psychopharmacology*, 15: 273–81.

Fox, H., Turner, J.J.D. and Parrott, A.C. (2001b) 'Dose related deficits in Rey's Auditory Verbal Learning Task, in abstinent Ecstasy/MDMA users', *Human Psychopharmacology*, 16: 615–20.

Freeman, W.J. (1999) *How Brains Make Up their Minds*, London: Phoenix, Orion Press.

Freud, S. (1923) 'The ego and the id', in *Standard Edition*, vol. 19. London: Hogarth Press.

Gabbard, G.O. (2000) 'Disguise or consent', *International Journal of Psychoanalysis*, 81 (6): 1071–86.

Gallagher, S. and Meltzoff, A.N. (1996) 'The earliest sense of self and others: Merleau-Ponty and recent developmental studies', *Philosophical Psychology*, 9: 211–33.

Gallese, V., Fadiga, L., Fogassi, L. and Rizzolatti, G. (2002) 'Action representation and the inferior parietal lobule', in W. Prinz and B. Hommel (eds) *Common Mechanisms in Perception and Action: Attention and performance*, vol. 19: 334–55, New York: Oxford University Press.

Gamwell, L. (2000) 'The muse is within: the psyche in a century of science', in L. Gamwell (ed.) *Dreams 1900–2000: Science, art and the unconscious mind*, Ithaca, NY: Cornell University Press.

Gerhardt, S. (2004) *Why Love Matters: How affection shapes a baby's brain*, Hove and New York: Brunner-Routledge.

Gogtay, N., Giedd, J.N., Lusk, L., Hayashi, K.M., Greenstein, D., Vaituzis, A.C., Nugent III, T.F., Herman, D.H., Clasen, L.S., Toga, A.W., Rapaport, J.L. and Thompson, P.M. (2004) 'Dynamic mapping of human cortical development during childhood through early adulthood', *Proceedings of the National Academy of Sciences USA*, 101 (21): 8174–9.

Goldberg, E. (2001) *The Executive Brain: Frontal lobes and the civilised mind*, Oxford and New York: Oxford University Press.

Goodwin, J. (2002) 'Snow White and the seven diagnoses', in V. Sinason (ed.) *Attachment, Trauma and Multiplicity: Working with dissociative identity disorder*, Hove: Brunner-Routledge.

Green, V. (2003) *Emotional Development in Psychoanalysis, Attachment Theory and Neuroscience: Creating connections*, Hove and New York: Brunner-Routledge.

Grillon, C., Southwick, S.M. and Charney, D.S. (1996) 'The psychobiological basis of post-traumatic stress disorder', *Molecular Psychiatry*, 1: 278–97.

Hamer, D. (2002) 'Genetics: rethinking behavior genetics', *Science*, 298 (5591): 71–2.

Hariri, A.R., Bookheimer, S.Y. and Mazziotta, J.C. (2000) 'Modulating emotional responses: effects of a neocortical network on the limbic system', *Neuroreport*, 11 (1): 43–8.

Harper, C.C. and McLanahan, S.S. (2004) 'Father absence and youth incarceration', *Journal of Research on Adolescence*, 14 (3): 369–97.

Hartmann, E. (2000) 'The psychology and physiology of dreaming: a new synthesis', in L. Gamwell (ed.) *Dreams 1900–2000: Science, art and the unconscious mind*, Ithaca, NY: Cornell University Press.

Hebb, D.O. (1949) *Organisation and behaviour*, New York: Wiley.

Heilman, K.M., Barrett, A.M. and Adair, J.C. (1998) 'Possible mechanisms of anosognosia: a defect in self-awareness', *Philosophical Transactions of Royal Society, London B*, 353: 1903–9.

Herzog, J.M. (1980) 'Sleep disturbance and father hunger in 18 to 28-month-old boys: the Erlkonig syndrome', *Psychoanalytic Study of the Child*, 35: 219–33.

Hillman, J. and McLean, M. (1997) *Dream Animals*, San Francisco, CA: Chronicle.

Hobson, J.A. (1999) 'The new neuropsychology of sleep: implications for psychoanalysis', *Neuropsychoanalysis*, 1 (2): 157–83.

Hobson, J.A. and Pace-Schott, E.F. (1999) 'Response to commentaries on the new neuropsychology of sleep: implications for neuropsychoanalysis', *Neuropsychoanalysis*, 1 (2): 206–24.

Holmes, J. (1996) *Attachment, Intimacy, Autonomy: Using attachment theory in adult psychotherapy*, Northvale, NJ: Aronson.

Hopkins, J. (1986) 'Solving the mystery of monsters: steps towards the recovery from trauma', *Journal of Child Psychotherapy*, 12 (1): 61–71.

Horgan, J. (1999) 'Can science explain consciousness?', in *The Scientific American Book of the Brain*, Guilford, CT: Lyons Press.

Houdé, O., Zago, L., Crivello, F., Moutier, S., Pineau, A., Mazoyer, B. and Tzourio-Mazoyer, N. (2001) 'Access to deductive logic depends on a right ventromedial prefrontal area devoted to emotion and feeling: evidence from a training paradigm', *NeuroImage*, 14: 1486–92.

Jacoby, M. (1969) 'A contribution to the phenomenon of transference', *Journal of Analytical Psychology*, 14 (2): 133–42.

Janet, P. (1889) *L'Automatisme psychologique*, Paris: Alcan.

Johnson, S.C. (2000) 'The recognition of mentalistic agents in infancy', *Trends in Cognitive Science*, 4: 22–8.

Johnson and Johnson Services Inc. Video (2000) *Amazing Talents of the Newborn*, New York: Johnson and Johnson Pediatric Institute, LLC.

Joseph, R. (1992) *The Right Brain and the Unconscious: Discovering the stranger within*, New York: Plenum Press.

Jung, C.G. (1904) 'Studies in word association', *CW* 2.

—— (1912) 'The theory of psychoanalysis', *CW* 4.

—— (1928) 'The therapeutic value of abreaction', *CW* 16: para. 267.

—— (1934a) 'A review of the complex theory', *CW* 8: paras. 200–3.

—— (1934b) 'The meaning of psychology for modern man', *CW* 10.

—— (1935) *The Tavistock Lectures*, *CW* 18.

—— (1938) *Terry Lectures*, Yale University, New Haven, CT; published in *CW* 11: para. 41.

—— (1946) 'Analytical psychology and education', *CW* 17: para. 189.

—— (1953a) 'Individual dream symbolism in relation to alchemy', *CW* 12: para. 44.

—— (1953b) 'The relations between the Ego and the unconscious', *CW* 7: para. 274.

—— (1954a) 'The practical use of dream-analysis', *CW* 16.

—— (1954b) 'The significance of the unconscious in individual education', *CW* 17: para. 260.

—— (1954c) 'The development of personality', *CW* 17: paras. 317–21.

—— (1954d) 'Child development and education', *CW* 17.

Jung, C.G. (1960) 'General aspects of dream psychology', *CW* 8: para. 509.

—— (1962) *Memories, Dreams, Reflections*, recorded by A. Jaffé (ed.), New York: Pantheon; London: Collins and Routledge and Kegan Paul; paperback edition, London: Fontana.

Kagan, R. (2004) *Rebuilding Attachments with Traumatized Children*, New York: Haworth Press.

Kalsched, D. (1996) *The Inner World of Trauma: Archetypal defences of the human spirit*, London and New York: Routledge.

—— (1999) 'Response to "The multiple self: working with dissociation and trauma"', *Journal of Analytical Psychology*, 44 (4): 465–74.

Kaplan-Solms, K. and Solms, M. (2000) *Clinical Studies in Neuro-Psychoanalysis: Introduction to a depth neuropsychology*, Madison, CT: International Universities Press.

Khan, M.R. (1971) ' "To hear with eyes": clinical notes on body as subject and object', in M.R. Khan, *The Privacy of the Self*, New York: International Universities Press; London: Hogarth Press.

Kirsch, T.B. (1968) 'The relationship of the REM state to analytical psychology', *American Journal of Psychiatry*, 124: 1459–63.

Knox, J. (2001) 'Memories, fantasies, archetypes: an exploration of some connections between cognitive science and analytical psychology', *Journal of Analytical Psychology*, 46 (4): 613–35.

—— (2003) *Archetype, Attachment, Analysis: Jungian psychology and the emergent mind*, London: Brunner-Routledge.

—— (2004) 'Developmental aspects of analytical psychology: new perspectives from cognitive science and attachment theory – Jung's model of the mind', in J. Cambray and L. Carter (eds) *Analytical Psychology: Contemporary perspectives in Jungian analysis*, Hove and New York: Brunner-Routledge.

Lakoff, G. and Johnson, M. (1999) *Philosophy in the Flesh: The embodied mind and its challenge to western thought*, New York: Basic Books.

Lanius, R., Williamson, P.C., Densmore, M., Boksman, K., Neufeld, R.W., Gati, J.S. and Menon, R. (2004) 'The nature of traumatic memories: a 4-T fMRI functional connectivity analysis', *American Journal of Psychiatry*, 161: 36–44.

Lanyado, M. (1999) 'Traumatization in children', in M. Lanyado and A. Horne (eds) *The Handbook of Child and Adolescent Psychotherapy*, London: Routledge.

LeDoux, J.E. (1996) *The Emotional Brain*, New York: Simon and Schuster.

—— (1999) 'Emotion, memory and the brain', in *The Scientific American Book of the Brain*, Guilford, CT: Lyons Press.

—— (2002) *Synaptic Self: How our brains become who we are*, London: Pan Macmillan.

Legerstee, M. (1991) 'The role of the person and object in eliciting early imitation', *Journal of Experimental Child Psychology*, 51: 423–33.

Levin, F. (1997) 'Integrating some mind and brain views of transference: the phenomena', *Journal of the American Psychoanalytic Association*, 45: 1121–52.

Levine, P. (1997) *Waking the Tiger: Healing trauma*, Berkeley, CA: North Atlantic Books.

Ludlow, C.L. (2000) 'Stuttering: dysfunction in a complex and dynamic system', *Brain*, 123: 1983–4.

Luria, A.R. (1987) 'Mind and brain: Luria's philosophy', in R.L. Gregory (ed.) *The Oxford Companion to the Mind*, Oxford and New York: Oxford University Press.

McCann, I.L. and Colletti, J. (1994) 'The dance of empathy: a hermeneutic formulation of countertransference, empathy and understanding in individuals who have experienced early childhood trauma', in J.P. Wilson and J. Lindy (eds) *Countertransference in the Treatment of PTSD*, New York and London: Guilford Press.

McDougall, J. (1989) *Theatres of the Body: A psychoanalytical approach to psychosomatic illness*, London: Free Association Books.

Mandler, J.M. and McDonough, L. (2000) 'Advancing downward to the basic level', *Journal of Cognition and Development*, 1: 379–403.

Marvin, R., Cooper, G., Hoffman, K. and Powell, B. (2002) 'The circle of security project: attachment-based intervention with care-giver-pre-school child dyads', *Attachment and Human Development*, 4 (1): 107–24.

Meltzer, D.M. (1973) *Sexual States of Mind*, Strath Tay: Clunie Press.

Meltzoff, A.N. (1995) 'Understanding the intentions of others: re-enactment of intended acts by 18-month-old children', *Developmental Psychology*, 31: 838–50.

Meltzoff, A.N. and Moore, M.K. (1995) 'Infants' understanding of people and things: from body imitation to folk psychology', in J. Bermudez, A.J. Marcel and N. Eilan (eds) *Body and the Self*, Cambridge, MA: MIT Press.

Miller, A. (2005) *The Body Never Lies: The lingering effects of cruel parenting*, New York and London: Norton.

Miller, G. (2004) 'Forgetting and remembering: learning to forget', *Science*, 304 (5667): 34–6.

Milne, A.A. (1958 [1926]) *Winnie-the-Pooh*, London: Methuen.

Mitrani, J.L. (2001) *Ordinary People and Extra-ordinary Protections: A Post-Kleinian approach to the treatment of primitive mental states*, Hove: Brunner-Routledge; Philadelphia, PA: Taylor and Francis.

Modell, A.H. (1997) 'Reflections on metaphors and affects', *Annual of Psychoanalysis*, 25: 219–33.

—— (1999) 'The dead mother syndrome and the reconstruction of trauma', in *The Dead Mother*, The New Library of Psychoanalysis, London: Routledge.

Mollon, P. (1996) *Multiple Selves, Multiple Voices*, Chichester: Wiley.

—— (2002) 'Dark dimensions of multiple personality', in V. Sinason (ed.) *Attachment, Trauma and Multiplicity: Working with dissociative identity disorder*, Hove: Brunner-Routledge.

Morgan, M. (2002) 'Ecstasy: throwing the baby out with the bath water?', *The Psychologist*, 15 (9): 468–9.

Morton, J. and Johnson, M.H. (1991) 'CONSPEC and CONLEARN: a two-process theory of infant face recognition', *Psychological Review*, 98: 164–81.

Myers, C.S. (1940) *Shell Shock in France 1914–1918*, Cambridge: Cambridge University Press.

Naccache, L., Gaillard, R., Adam, C., Hasboun, D., Clémenceau, S., Baulac, M., Dehaene, S. and Cohen, L. (2005) 'A direct intracranial record of emotions evoked by subliminal words', *Proceedings of the National Academy of Sciences USA*, 102 (21): 7713–17.

Nakamura, K., Kawashima, R., Ito, K., Sugiura, M., Kato, T., Nakamura, A. et al. (1999) 'Activation of the right inferior frontal cortex during assessment of facial emotion', *Journal of Neurophysiology*, 82: 1610–14.

Nijenhuis, E.R.S. and Van der Hart, O. (1999) 'Forgetting and reexperiencing trauma', in J. Goodwin, J. Attias and R. Attias (eds) *Splintered Reflections: Images of the body in trauma*, New York: Basic Books.

Nijenhuis, E.R.S., Van der Hart, O. and Steele, K. (2004) 'Trauma-related structural dissociation of the personality', Trauma Information Pages Website, January 2004: http://www.trauma-pages.com/Nijenhuis–2004.htm

O'Brien, G. and Opie, J. (2003) 'The multiplicity of consciousness and the emergence of the Self', in T. Kircher and A. David (eds) *The Self in Neuroscience and Psychiatry*, Cambridge: Cambridge University Press.

Ochsner, K.N., Bunge, S.A., Gross, J.J. and Gabrieli, J.D. (2002) 'Rethinking feelings: an FMRI study of the cognitive regulation of emotion', *Journal of Cognitive Neuroscience*, 14 (8): 1215–29.

Pally, R. (2000) *The Mind–Brain Relationship*, London and New York: Karnac.

Panksepp, J. (1998) *Affective Neuroscience: The foundations of human and animal emotions*, New York and Oxford: Oxford University Press.

—— (2003) 'The neural nature of the core SELF: implications for understanding schizophrenia', in T. Kircher and A. David (eds) *The Self in Neuroscience and Psychiatry*, Cambridge: Cambridge University Press.

Parrott, A. (2002) 'Ecstasy: very real, very damaging', *The Psychologist*, 15: 472–3.

Paus, T. (2005) 'Mapping brain maturation and cognitive development during adolescence', *Trends in Cognitive Sciences*, 9 (2): 60–8.

Paus, T., Zijdenbos, A., Worsley, K., Collins, D.L., Blumenthal, J., Giedd, J.N., Rappaport, J.L. and Evans, A.C. (1999) 'Structural maturation of neural pathways in children and adolescents: in vivo study', *Science*, 283: 1908–11.

Perry, B.D. (1999) 'The memories of states: how the brain stores and retrieves experience', in J.M. Goodwin and R. Attias (eds) *Splintered Reflections: Images of the body in trauma*, New York: Basic Books.

Perry, B.D., Pollard, R.A., Blakley, T.L., Baker, E.W.L. and Vigilante, D. (1995) 'Childhood trauma, the neurobiology of adaptation, and "use-dependent" development of the brain: how "states" become "traits"', *Infant Mental Health Journal*, 16 (4): 271–91.

Porges, S.W. (1996) 'Emotion: an evolutionary by-product of the neural regulation of the autonomic nervous system', in C.S. Carter, B. Kirkpatrick and I.I. Lederhendler (eds) *The Integrative Neurobiology of Affiliation*, New York: Annals of the New York Academy of Sciences.

Post, R.M. and Weiss, S.R.B. (1998) 'Sensitisation and kindling in mood, anxiety, and obsessive-compulsive disorders: the role of serotinergic mechanisms in illness progression', *Biological Psychiatry*, 44 (3): 193–206.

Putnam, F.W. (1997) *Dissociation in Children and Adolescents: A developmental perspective*, New York: Guilford Press.

Quinodoz, J.-M. (2002) *Dreams that Turn Over a Page: Paradoxical dreams in psychoanalysis*, London: Brunner-Routledge.

Redfearn, J.W.T. (1985) *My Self, My Many Selves*, London: Academic Press.

Reinders, A.A.T.S., Nijenhuis, E.R.S., Paans, A.M.J., Korf, J., Willemsen, A.T.M. and den Boor, J.A. (2003) 'One brain, two selves', *Neuroimage*, 20: 2119–25.

Reiser, M.F. (1999) 'Commentary on the new neuropsychology of sleep', *Neuropsychoanalysis*, 1 (2): 196–206.

Restak, R. (2001) *The Secret Life of the Brain*, Washington, DC: National Academy Press.

Ribeiro, S. (2004) 'Towards an evolutionary theory of sleep and dreams', *MultiCiência*, 3.

Ricaurte, G.A., DeLanney, L.E., Irwin, I. and Langston, J.W. (1988) 'Toxic effects of 3,4-methylenedioxymeth-amphetamine (MDMA) on central serotonergic neurons in the primate: importance of route and frequency of drug administration', *Brain Research*, 446: 165–8.

Rizzolatti, G., Fadiga, L., Fogassi, L. and Gallese, V. (1999) 'Resonance behaviours and mirror neurons', *Archives of Italian Biology*, 137: 85–100.

Rochat, P. (ed.) (1999) *Early Social Cognition: Understanding others in the first months of Life*, Mahwah, NJ: Erlbaum.

Rochat, P. and Hespos, S.J. (1997) 'Differential rooting response by neonates: evidence for an early sense of self', *Early Development and Parenting*, 6: 105–12.

Rosen, J.B. and Schulkin, J. (1998) 'From normal fear to pathological anxiety', *Psychological Review*, 105 (2): 325–50.

Rosenbaum, T. (2002) *The Golems of Gotham*, New York: HarperCollins.

Rossi, E.L. (2004) 'Sacred spaces and places in healing dreams: gene expression and brain growth in rehabilitation', *Psychological Perspectives*, 47 (1): 48–63.

Rothschild, B. (2000) *The Body Remembers: The psychobiology of trauma and trauma treatment*, New York: Norton.

Rowling, J.K. (1997) *Harry Potter and the Philosopher's Stone*, London: Bloomsbury.

Scaer, R.C. (2001a) *The Body Bears the Burden: Trauma, dissociation and disease*, New York, London and Oxford: Haworth Press.

—— (2001b) 'The neurophysiology of dissociation and chronic disease', *Applied Psychology and Biofeedback*, 26 (1): 73–91.

Schank, R.C. (1999) *Dynamic Memory Revisited*, Cambridge and New York: Cambridge University Press.

Schank, R.C. and Morson, G.S. (1990) *Tell Me a Story: Narrative and intelligence*, Evanston, IL: Northwestern University Press.

Schore, A.N. (1994) *Affect Regulation and the Origin of the Self: The neurobiology of emotional development*, Hillsdale, NJ: Erlbaum.

—— (1996) 'The experience-dependent maturation of a regulatory system in the orbital prefrontal cortex and the origin of developmental psychopathology', *Development and Psychopathology*, 8: 59–87.

—— (2001a) 'Minds in the making: attachment – the self-organising brain and developmentally-oriented psychoanalytic psychotherapy', *British Journal of Psychotherapy*, 17 (3): 299–328.

—— (2001b) 'The right brain as the neurobiological substratum of Freud's dynamic unconscious', in D. Scharff (ed.) *The Psychoanalytic Century: Freud's legacy for the future*, New York: Other Press.

—— (2001c) 'The effects of relational trauma on right brain development, affect regulation, and infant mental health', *Infant Mental Health Journal*, 22: 210–69.

—— (2002) 'Dysregulation of the right brain: a fundamental mechanism of traumatic attachment and the psychopathogenesis of posttraumatic stress disorder', *Australian and New Zealand Journal of Psychiatry*, 36 (1): 9–30.

—— (2003a) *Affect Dysregulation and Disorders of the Self*, New York: Norton.

—— (2003b) *Affect Regulation and Repair of the Self*, New York: Norton.

—— (in press) 'Attachment trauma and the developing right brain: origins of pathological dissociation', in *Dissociation and Dissociative Disorders DSM-5 and Beyond*.

Searles, H. (1986) *My Work with Borderline Patients*, Northvale, NJ: Aronson.

Segal, H. (1991) *Dream, Art, Phantasy*, London and New York: Routledge.

Sherwood, D. (2006) Response to M. Wilkinson's paper 'The Dreaming Mind-Brain', *Journal of Analytical Psychology*, 51, 1.

Shin, Y.-W., Lee, J.-S., Han, O.-S. and Rih, B.-Y. (2005) 'The influence of complexes on implicit learning', *Journal of Analytical Psychology*, 50 (2): 175–90.

Sidoli, M. (2000) *When the Body Speaks: The archetypes in the body*, ed. P. Blakemore, London and Philadelphia, PA: Routledge.

Siegel, D. (1999) *The Developing Mind: Toward a neurobiology of inter-personal experience*, New York: Guilford Press.

—— (2003) 'An interpersonal neurobiology of psychotherapy', in M.F. Solomon and D.J. Siegel (eds) *Healing Trauma: Attachment, mind, body and brain*, New York and London: Norton.

Sieratzki, J.S. and Woll, B. (1996) 'Why do mothers cradle babies on their left?', *Lancet*, 347: 1746–8.

Sinason, V. (2002) 'The shoemaker and the elves: working with multiplicity', in V. Sinason (ed.) *Attachment, Trauma and Multi-plicity: Working with dissociative identity disorder*, Hove: Brunner-Routledge.

Solms, M. (1999) 'Commentary on the new neuropsychology of sleep', *Neuropsychoanalysis*, 1 (2): 183–95.

Solms, M. and Greenfield, S. (2002) 'The private life of the brain dialogue' in the *On the Way Home* series, Institute of Psychoanalysis, London, 30 October.

Solms, M. and Turnbull, O. (2002) *The Brain and the Inner World: An introduction to the neuroscience of subjective relationship*, New York: Other Press.

Solomon, H.M. (1998) 'The self in transformation: the passage from a two- to a three-dimensional internal world', *Journal of Analytical Psychology*, 43 (2): 225–38.

—— (2004) 'Self creation and the "as if" personality', *Journal of Analytical Psychology*, 49 (5): 635–56.

Spiegel, D. and Cardena, E. (1991) 'Disintegrated experience: the dissocia-tive disorders revisited', *Journal of Abnormal Psychology*, 100: 366–78.

Stein, L. (1967) 'Introducing not-self', *Journal of Analytical Psychology*, 12 (2): 97–113.

Stern, D. (1985) *The Interpersonal World of the Infant*, New York: Basic Books.

Stewart, H. (1992) *Psychic Experience and Problems of Technique*, London and New York: Routledge.

Stolorow, R. (1997) 'Principles of dynamic systems, intersubjectivity, and the obsolete distinction between one-person and two-person psychologies', *Psychoanalytic Dialogues*, 7: 859–68.

Sullivan, R.M. and Gratton, A. (2002) 'Prefrontal cortical regulation of hypothalamic-pituitary-adrenal function in the rat and implications for psychopathology: side matters', *Psychoneuroendocrinology*, 27: 99–114.

Symington, J. (1985) 'The survival function of primitive omnipotence', *International Journal of Psychoanalysis*, 66: 481–8.

Taylor, E. (1982) *William James on Exceptional Mental States: The 1896 Lowell Lectures*, New York: Scribners.

Teicher, M. (2000) 'Wounds that time won't heal: the neurobiology of child abuse', *Cerebrum*, 2 (4): 50–67.

—— (2002) 'Scars that will not heal: the neurobiology of child abuse', *Scientific American*, 286 (3): 68–75.

Terr, L.C. (1991) 'Childhood traumas: an outline and overview', *American Journal of Psychiatry*, 148 (1): 322–34.

—— (1994) 'True memories of childhood trauma: flaws, absences and returns', in *The Recovered Memory/False Memory Debate*, London: Academic Press.

Trevarthen, C. (1989) 'Development of early social interactions and the affective regulations of brain growth', in C. von Euler and H. Forssberg (eds) *The Neurobiology of Early Infant Behaviour*, New York: Macmillan.

Tronick, E. (1998) 'Dyadically expanded states of consciousness and the process of therapeutic change', *Infant Mental Health Journal*, 44: 290–9.

Trowell, J. (1998) 'Child sexual abuse and gender identity development: some understanding from work with girls who have been sexually abused', in D. Di Ceglie and D. Freedman (eds) *A Stranger in my Own Body*, London: Karnac.

Tzourio-Mazoyer, N., DeSchonen, S., Crivello, F., Reutter, B., Aujard, S. and Mazoyer, B. (2002) 'Neural correlates of woman face processing by 2-month-old infants', *NeuroImage*, 15: 451–61.

van der Kolk, B.A. (1996) 'The body keeps the score: approaches to the psychobiology of posttraumatic stress disorder', in B.A. van der Kolk, A.C. McFarlane and L. Weisaeth (eds) *Traumatic Stress: The effects of overwhelming experience on mind, body and society*, New York and London: Guilford Press.

—— (2000) 'Post traumatic stress disorder and the nature of trauma', *Dialogues in Clinical Neuroscience*, 2 (1): 7–22.

Watt, D.E. (2005) 'Social bonds and the nature of empathy', *Journal of Consciousness Studies*, 12 (8–10): 185–209.

Westen, D. and Gabbard, O.G. (2002) 'Cognitive neuroscience, conflict and compromise', *Journal of the American Psychoanalytic Association*, 50 (1): 53–98.

Wilkinson, M.A. (2001) 'His mother tongue: from stuttering to separation, a case history', *Journal of Analytical Psychology*, 46 (2): 257–74.

—— (2003) 'Undoing trauma: contemporary neuroscience – a clinical perspective', *Journal of Analytical Psychology*, 48 (2): 235–53.

—— (2004) 'The mind-brain relationship: the emergent self', *Journal of Analytical Psychology*, 49 (1): 83–101.

—— (2005) 'Undoing dissociation: affective neuroscience – a contemporary Jungian clinical perspective', *Journal of Analytical Psychology*, 50 (4): 483–501.

—— (2006) 'The dreaming mind-brain, a Jungian perspective', *Journal of Analytical Psychology*.

Williams, G.P. (2004) Response to Dr Barry Proner's paper 'Bodily states of anxiety', given at the Scientific Meeting of the Society of Analytical Psychology, London, 4 October.

Williams, L. (1994) 'Recall of childhood trauma: a prospective study of women's memories of childhood sexual abuse', *Journal of Consulting and Clinical Psychology*, 62: 1167–76.

Winnicott, D.W. (1960) 'True and false self', in D.W. Winnicott (ed.) (1965) *The Maturational Process and the Facilitating Environment*, London: Hogarth Press.

—— (1965) *The Maturational Process and the Facilitating Environment*, London: Hogarth Press.

Woodhead, J. (2004) ' "Dialectical process" and "constructive method": micro-analysis of relational process in an example from parent–infant psychotherapy', *Journal of Analytical Psychology*, 49 (2): 143–60.

—— (2005) 'Shifting triangles: images of father in sequences from parent–infant psychotherapy', *International Journal of Infant Observation*, 7 (2–3): 76–90.

World Health Organization (WHO) (1992) *The ICD-10 Classification of Mental and Behavioural Disorders*, Geneva: WHO.

Yehuda, R. (1998) *Psychological Trauma*, Washington, DC and London: American Psychiatric Press.

Yurgelun-Todd, D. (1998) 'Brain and psyche: the neurobiology of the self', paper presented at the 'Brain and Psyche' seminar at the Whitehead Institute for Biomedical Research, Cambridge, MA.

Zakanis, K.K. and Young, D.A. (2001) 'Memory impairment in abstinent MDMA (Ecstasy) users: a longitudinal investigation', *Neurology*, 56: 966–9.

Zeki, S. and Bartels, A. (1998) 'The asynchrony of consciousness', *Proceedings of the Royal Society of London*, 265: 1583–5.

Index